Break
the Cycle of
ALCOHOLISM

Skills for
Healthy Sobriety

To my wife Nola

> Who can find a good woman? She is precious beyond all things.
>
> PROV. 31:10
>
> Geoff Colvin

To my brother Dan who has always been there for me, whose quiet humor helps me gain perspective.

> Bob Wiese

To my family, my support

> Tina Wells

Break the Cycle of ALCOHOLISM

Skills for Healthy Sobriety

Geoff Colvin | Bob Wiese | Tina Wells

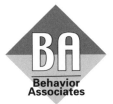

BA

Behavior Associates

For information:
Behavior Associates
2585 Windsor Circle East
Eugene, Oregon, 97405
(541) 485-6450
Fax: (541) 344-9680
www.behaviorassociates.org

Printed in United States of America
Geoff Colvin (Geoffrey Thomas Colvin), 1941–
Bob Wiese (Robert John Wiese), 1940–
Tina Wells, (Tina Cranor Wells), 1956–
Break the cycle of alcoholism: Skills for healthy sobriety
Includes bibliographical references and index.
ISBN 978-0-9631777-5-9

Cover design, graphic design, book design, and production: *Kylee Lee*
Index: *Catharyn Martz*

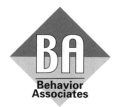

About the Authors

Geoff Colvin, PhD, Senior Author, has worked as a behavior consultant, certified school psychologist, teacher and school administrator, and researcher at University of Oregon. He is nationally and internationally recognized as a leader in the field of working with individuals who have severe behavior problems. In 2011 he delivered the keynote address for the 50th Anniversary International Conference celebration for the Council for Children with Behavior Disorders in New Orleans. In 2010 he received the Northwest Positive Behavior and Intervention Supports (PBIS) Inaugural Life Time Achievement Award. Colvin is a talented and successful author of books, chapters, monographs, professional journal articles, and DVD/video programs for professional development. He regularly presents keynotes nationally and internationally. His grant-funded research activities include a 2008–2009 position as principal investigator for a National Institute of Health grant on safety in the workplace titled Alcohol Servers Applying Psychology (ASAP). He has also contributed articles to the Emerald Valley Intergroup (the coordinating agency for Alcoholics Anonymous in Lane County, Oregon).

Bob Wiese began his career as a high school English literature teacher and moved to teaching students with severe behavior problems in a specialized program directed by Colvin. He has served in many roles with Alcoholics Anonymous for the past 25 years. He has been, and still is, a highly involved sponsor supporting numerous recovering alcoholics, especially those in their early days of sobriety. He provides training at a state level for counselors of alcoholics and has provided in-service and delivered lectures on alcoholism in many settings throughout the Northwest. He shows a keen insight into the problems alcoholics face and provides helpful roadmaps for recovering alcoholics to achieve sobriety, remain sober, and engage in productive lives.

Tina Wells, editor and author, has worked directly with Colvin on several of his published books, including *Managing the Cycle of Acting-Out Behavior in the Classroom* and *7 Steps for Developing A Proactive Schoolwide Discipline Plan.* She has been a Direct Instruction editor for numerous SRA-McGraw/Hill publications and currently edits books for the International Society for Technology in Education. She enjoys linguistics and harp. She has authored and coauthored various books ranging from spelling books (in English, *SRA Spelling Mastery,* and Japanese, *Easy Katakana: How to Read and Write English Words Used in Japanese*) to music books for harps and lyres.

Acknowledgments

We wish to thank the following people who took the time to read our manuscript in the development phase and for providing us with valuable feedback: Mike M., Linda C., Bob D., Paul M., and Jerry G.

We are grateful to Brenda Cervantes for providing us with a wonderful venue for our weekly meetings at Gary's (Brenda's memorial coffee shop in honor of her late son Gary). Also our thanks are due to John Crane for his gracious service.

We are especially appreciative of Linda Carnine and Jerry Gjesvold for their careful reading of the manuscript, their excellent feedback, and very helpful contributions.

Scott Whitehead deserves our thanks for his highly skilled technical computer support in the writing of the manuscript.

Our special thanks are due to Kylee Lee who generated the graphics for this book. She was able to translate our general ideas into very helpful and lucid diagrams and figures.

Contents

Introduction

Alcoholism has been and still is one of the most serious social problems facing society today, not only in America, but throughout the world. The numbers affected by alcoholism are vast and the effects of the problem significantly impact every level of humanity and every corner of our culture. Billions of dollars have been spent over many years to research the subject, address the issues, treat the victims, and pay for the repercussions of excessive on-going drinking. Understandably, much has been written on the subject of alcoholism to describe the problems, analyze the causes, and prescribe solutions. Moreover, there is a wealth of information, programs, agencies, and services readily available to individuals, families, caretakers, and institutions to provide high levels of support and assistance.

Why then should another book be written on this subject? In this book the problem of alcoholism is addressed from the perspective of *behavioral psychology*. This approach has two main steps when it comes to addressing problem behavior. First is *behavioral analysis* in which the various factors contributing to the problem behavior are identified with the intent of understanding how the behavior is developed and maintained. The second step involves establishing new and acceptable replacement behaviors through the teaching and learning process of skill development. Behavioral psychology has been the subject of research and practices for decades in many human service agencies such as public schools, prisons, mental health institutions, residential care facilities for disturbed children and adults, and prisons. Providers in these agencies—educators, psychologists, counselors, law enforcement personnel, and support professionals have benefited from the huge body of literature available on this research, best practice procedures, and descriptions of effective strategies for managing children and adults who exhibit serious problem behavior.

It is not a big stretch to apply these same behavioral analyses and skill development interventions to address the habitual problem behavior of alcoholism. The reason is that we are dealing with human behavior. While the settings and circumstances may vary, the principles for dealing with human behavior do not change. This is because human beings act in relatively predictable ways and patterns. The challenge is to adapt and apply this approach of behavioral psychology to the unique features of alcoholism.

This book is designed to take the principles and practices of behavioral psychology and *apply* them to the subject of alcoholism. It is expected that this approach will assist those afflicted with alcoholism and offer service providers in the field with a deeper *understanding* of the tragic phenomenon of alcoholism, strengthen their ability to break up the patterns of alcoholism, and establish and maintain new skills for lifelong healthy recovery. This model basically depicts competing options for alcoholics in terms of pathways. One pathway leads to chronic alcoholism and the second one, the replacement pathway, leads to beginning sobriety and ultimately to *healthy sobriety*. This book is designed to help alcoholics select and sustain practices for forging a pathway to a lifelong, healthy, sober lifestyle.

There are four sections in this book. The purpose of the first section, *Critical Perspectives*, is to provide important background information for understanding the problem of alcoholism. Chapter 1 gives background information on key issues of alcoholism. Chapter 2 presents a behavioral model which describes the phases of alcoholism from where an individual starts using alcohol for any number of reasons and gradual dependency on alcohol develops into alcoholism. Chapter 3 systematically examines the dynamics individuals face in making a firm commitment to confront and change their dependence on alcohol. It is understood that progress in effectively addressing alcoholism will not be long lasting without such a firm commitment.

The next two sections center on tools to be used in becoming sober and the skills to be developed once initial sobriety has been attained. Tools focus on strategies that are basically standard procedures in the field for becoming sober. Skills to be developed for healthy sobriety are more individualized and need to be maintained or developed for life.

The second section, *Tools for Beginning Sobriety,* is devoted to an explanation and description of the necessary steps needed to effectively disrupt the cycle of alcoholism and facilitate sobriety. Chapter 4, Tools for Detoxification, describes the universal first step toward breaking up the chemical dependence on alcohol. This process describes the tools needed to achieve alcohol cessation and manage the side effects of alcohol withdrawal. In Chapter 5, Tools for Defusing Cravings, information is presented on the nature of cravings and details on tools for effectively controlling these cravings. Chapter 6, Tools for Meeting Initial Needs, describes how tools adapted from *behavioral psychology* are applied to help alcoholics and their support people understand and identify the very factors that led to excessive alcohol use in the first place. The approach is to create an alternative pathway from alcoholism by re-tooling the recovering alcoholics so that needs are met in healthy ways rather than through the use of alcohol.

Section Three, *Skills for Healthy Sobriety,* is devoted to ongoing steps that need to be taken not only to maintain sobriety, a daunting challenge in itself, but to provide detailed information on the lifelong process of *skill development.* Individuals afflicted with alcoholism have experienced significant damage to their bodies and organs and substantial impairments to skills for normal functional living. A critical assumption in this book is that in order for recovering alcoholics to remain sober, they must not only *abstain from alcohol*, but they must become productively engaged in ongoing *skill development.* The section opens with Chapter 7, Key Considerations for Personal Growth, where central principles and guidelines are presented for helping recovering alcoholics develop the necessary skills in core human growth areas. In the next four chapters, detailed descriptions of interventions are presented for helping the recovering alcoholic to learn *lifelong skills* to foster healthy sobriety: Chapter 8: Skills for *Autonomous* Growth; Chapter 9: Skills for *Cognitive* Growth; Chapter 10: Skills for *Social* Growth; and Chapter 11: Skills for *Emotional* Growth.

The final section, Section Four: *Additional Considerations,* addresses topics that lie outside the desirable progression from understanding alcoholism, becoming sober, and developing skills to lead functional, sober, and healthy lives. Chapter 12: Addressing Relapse as Needed covers issues and procedures should the recovering alcoholic resume drinking. Though not a given it is understood that many alcoholics will relapse before attaining lifelong sobriety. Chapter 13: Frequently Asked Questions reviews common questions and issues raised by recovering alcoholics and their support personnel regarding the process of attaining and sustaining a healthy, sober lifestyle.

The majority of the chapters contain illustrations, forms, and checklists that have been designed to be used and individualized by the recovering alcoholic. The forms have been reproduced in the appendices at the end of this book for ongoing use as needed.

This book is written as a resource for persons involved with addressing alcoholism at a number of important levels:

- Professionals, such as physicians, therapists, counselors, psychologists, and social workers, in their work in helping their clients through the process of recovering from alcoholism to achieving healthy sobriety.

- Corrections staff involved in preparing incarcerated alcoholics and recovering alcoholics for their release and for parole officers monitoring and guiding them after release.

- Support people, such as sponsors, mentors, advisors, pastors, nurses, and friends who have a definite role in being present and helpful to alcoholics and in providing a roadmap for recovery.

- Family members, relatives, and significant others who have the complex responsibility and challenge of helping a loved one work through the problem of alcoholism and to understand what is involved.

- Recovering alcoholics who may use the tools described in this book and address the skills to be developed as a self-help guide in their quest for lifelong healthy sobriety. Recovering alcoholics come from all walks of life including clients, patients, persons in corrections, parolees, church members, employees across all occupations and careers, and loved ones—parents, siblings spouses, partners, significant others, and close friends.

SECTION ONE

Critical Perspectives

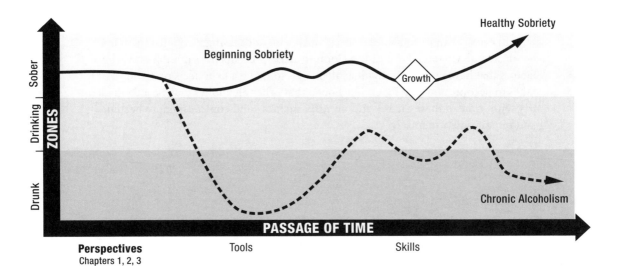

There is no question that alcoholism poses a very serious challenge to individuals, families, communities, and every level of society both nationally and internationally. Given that alcoholism is such a *complex* social problem, it is particularly important to address some key perspectives before any attempt is made to understand, describe, or propose interventions.

First, and foremost, it is crucial to ensure that the scope, gravity, and multiple issues of the problem of alcoholism are properly understood. In Chapter 1, The Problem of Alcoholism, key issues of alcoholism are discussed. The chapter is intended to highlight the enormity of the problem and to underscore the need to continually pursue interventions designed to assist afflicted individuals with recovery.

Secondly, there is no quick fix with interventions for alcoholism. If there were such a handy solution, the problems would not be so widespread, on going, and resistant to remediation. What is needed is a systematic model for understanding the various pieces that contribute to forming and maintaining alcoholism and, by implication, provide tools for remedying the problem and developing a sober lifestyle. In Chapter 2, Understanding the Pathway to Alcoholism, a model based on behavioral principles is presented to describe how alcoholism is established in the first place. This model will then be used in Sections Two and Three to frame interventions for developing and sustaining a quality life free of alcohol.

The third key perspective relates to the challenge of getting started. Unless there is buy-in, even the most fail-safe or surest means for addressing alcoholism will not be successful. Chapter 3, Making a Commitment, presents information on various factors that have enabled individual alcoholics to make a firm decision to do what it takes to become and stay sober. It is hoped that other alcoholics may be able to identify with some of these factors and, in turn, make a solid commitment to become and remain sober themselves.

The Problem of Alcoholism

1

Oh God, that men should put an enemy in their mouths to steal away their brains! That we should, with joy, pleasance, revel and applause, transform ourselves into beasts!

— Shakespeare, Othello

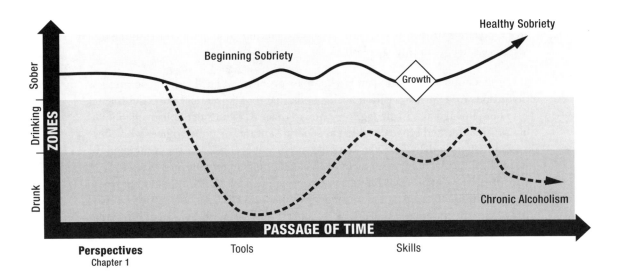

It is inarguable that alcoholism is a pervasive, life-threatening, destructive, and insidious problem for individuals, families, and society in general. The causes of alcoholism, its nature, and remedies have been the subject of research, varying practices, writings, and discussions for many decades.

The purpose of this chapter is to examine background information on alcoholism to ensure that there is some understanding of the complexity of the problem and awareness of current efforts and procedures for addressing these topics. It is beyond the scope of this book to take any of these topics to substantial depth. However, given the importance of this background information, additional resources are listed at the end of the chapter. The following topics related to alcoholism are addressed: 1. Definitions, 2. Risk factors, 3. Incidence, 4. Harmful effects, 5. Strategies and interventions, 6. Regulation of alcohol use, and 7. Trends.

Definitions

Definitions and descriptions of alcoholism are certainly plentiful in the literature. The pioneering work of E. Morton Jellinek and others argued for alcoholism to be treated as a disease with diagnoses and treatment based on physiological factors and levels. In a similar way, alcohol has been defined in terms of a drug and falls under the umbrella of drug addiction. There are issues as to the extent genetic factors contribute to the etiology and incidence of alcoholism. Some writers and researchers make discriminations based on levels of drinking in the form of a continuum from moderate drinking, to at-risk or binge drinking, to alcohol abuse, to the most serious cases of drinking, alcoholism.

It is understood that alcoholism is a complex problem and difficult to contain in a definition. We take the position in this book that for all practical purposes the field may be splitting hairs in struggling with language to define alcoholism, alcohol abuse, and repeated binge drinking as separate entities. A police officer who cites an individual for driving under the influence is not going to ask the individual if he or she is an alcoholic or an alcohol abuser. For example, the court, hearing a case of an individual who killed three people while driving drunk, does not pay too much attention to the particular category of the individual's alcoholism. The issue is whether the individual was drunk or sober. Similarly, with treatment programs there is not that much variability, if any, on interventions that are used for a person who is an alcoholic versus one who is a regular alcohol abuser.

For the purposes of this book, an operational or working description of alcoholism will be used based on features that can be readily identified and are directly related to outcomes of alcoholism. By using this approach we will be in a position to analyze alcoholism and develop interventions based on the principles of behavioral psychology, one of the cornerstones of this book. We define alcoholism in terms of three critical features or characteristics: dependency, inability to limit drinking, and inability to solve the problem alone.

Dependency. There exists a clear dependency on alcohol. The individual returns to excessive drinking on a regular basis. There is a clear pattern or cycle of drinking to excess in which the individual has a strong need, compulsion, or craving to drink. Alcohol has a grip so powerful a point is reached where the need to drink is uncontrollable.

Inability to Limit Drinking. Once the person starts drinking, he or she does not stop. The person gets on a roll and keeps drinking, finding creative ways to keep drinking once started. Some individuals can stop drinking for a period of time and then start up again. This person may or may not be alcoholic. However, alcoholic persons cannot, as a regular practice, limit themselves to two or three drinks. Once they start, they keep drinking to excess.

Inability to Solve the Problem Alone. Some individuals are able to address their problems with alcohol and develop and maintain plans for a life not controlled by alcohol. However, the vast majority of people with alcoholism need systematic help and support from others to be successful in maintaining sobriety. This assistance comes in the form of professional guidance, structure, and support from specialist organizations and agencies, and knowledgeable friends.

Risk Factors

We have chosen to use the term *risk factors* rather than causes or etiology of alcoholism. Risk factors suggest that the individual is more prone or more likely to become an alcoholic given the presence of these risk factors compared to individuals who are not exposed. Causes, on the other hand, may suggest that the individuals are victims in that they unwittingly become alcoholics because of the presence of these factors, similar to a person contracting malaria who is exposed to the disease-bearing mosquitoes. Causes, however, are likely to be critically important in medical analysis and some areas of psychosomatic research and corresponding development of treatment. Our approach, using behavioral psychology, is that there is a need to be cognizant of risk factors and these factors may need to be addressed in a recovery plan. Common risk factors include the following:

Genetic and Generational Alcoholism. Research shows that genetic factors can affect the way some individuals process and respond to alcohol. For example, the rate of alcoholism in men with no alcoholic parents is 11.4 percent while the rate is 29.5 percent for men with one alcoholic parent (http://mens-health.health-cares.net/alcoholism-risks.php).

Gender. Alcohol abuse is reported in the range of three to five times more frequent in men than in women. However, the incidence of alcoholism among women has risen significantly in recent decades (http://mens-health.health-cares.net/alcoholism-risks.php).

Associations. Individual drinking patterns can be influenced by the drinking practices of the people they associate with such as friends, relatives, work-mates, and the norms at parties and other gatherings or celebrations.

Psychological and Personality Factors. Some people are more prone to alcoholism because of their psychological or personality makeup. These people may be perfectionists, may have very high standards and low tolerance for frustration, may need high rates of support and encouragement at work or in relationships, and may have impulsive, aggressive, and reactive tendencies.

Cultural and Ethnic Factors. In some cultures alcohol use is very acceptable and is often the norm, such as in most western countries. In other cultures and religious groups, alcohol use is severely restricted. Research has shown some indigenous groups are particularly vulnerable to alcoholism (Saggers &

Gray, 1998). It has been reported that almost 12 percent of deaths through alcoholism occur among Native Americans and Alaska Natives. This is more than three times the rate of the general population (http://www.msnbc.msn.com/id/26439767/).

Age. Older people, especially at the onset of retirement, often show indications of higher alcohol consumption and, of course, have more opportunity or time to drink. In addition, younger people, especially adolescents, are more likely to engage in binge drinking as part of the risk-taking and peer pressure associated with growing up.

Mental Illness. Researchers have found high rates of alcohol use among individuals with mental health issues, especially anxiety disorders of depression, manic-depression, personality disorders, and schizophrenia (http://alcoholism.about.com/cs/dual/a/aa981209.htm).

Stress Management. Some people turn to alcohol use as a means of reducing stress. Stress can come in many different forms such as sudden changes in lifestyle and finances, business problems, relationship issues, and on-going sickness and death in the family.

Incidence

The statistics on incidence of alcoholism have been very well documented in our society and others for many decades. Given the considerable variability in defining alcoholism, we can expect a degree of variability in accuracy and in consistency of these measures. Regardless, the overall picture of the incidence of alcoholism, nationally and internationally, poses a very serious challenge to our society at every age group level and in all walks of life. Alcoholism has, in the past and certainly in the present, afflicted a staggering number of people. Some of the major statistics and trends are summarized in Box 1.1: A Statistics Summary of Alcoholism and Alcohol Abuse.

BOX 1.1: A Statistics Summary of Alcoholism and Alcohol Abuse

- Just under 13.8 million U.S. adults have issues with alcohol (approximately 1 in every 13 Americans), and 8.1 million of them officially suffer from alcoholism.

- An estimated 43% of U.S. adults have had someone related to them who is presently, or was, an alcoholic.

- 3 million U.S. citizens older than 60 abuse alcohol or require it to function normally.

- Alcohol abuse is 3–5 times more for males (9.8 million) than females (3.9 million).

- 6.6 million minors in the U.S. live with an alcoholic mother or father.

- Children of alcoholics are about four times more likely than the general population to develop alcohol problems.

- Generally, employees who have divorced, separated, or never married are twice as likely to have alcohol problems as those who are married. (Alcoholism Stats: www.treatment-centers.net/alcoholism-statistics.html)

- The younger you are when you start drinking, the greater your chance of becoming addicted to alcohol at some point in your life. More than 4 in 10 people who begin drinking before age 15 eventually become alcoholics. (National Institute on Alcohol Abuse and Alcoholism, 2003)

- Almost half of Americans aged 12 or older surveyed in 2001 reported being current drinkers of alcohol (48.3 percent or 109 million people).

- Both the rate of alcohol use and the number of drinkers increased steadily from 2000 to 2004.

- Current alcohol use remained steady among older age groups. (U.S. Department of Health and Human Services, 2002; www.oas.samhsa.gov/nhsda/2k1nhsda/vol1/Chapter3.htm)

Harmful Effects

The repercussions for alcoholism and alcohol abuse are very serious and, generally, quite devastating. In many cases, the results can be life-threatening. Heavy and uncontrolled drinking significantly increases the risk for several medical conditions and diseases such as cancers, especially those of the liver, esophagus, throat, and larynx (voice box). It can also cause liver cirrhosis, immune system problems, brain damage, and harm to the fetus during pregnancy. In addition, excessive drinking is substantially related to incidences of death from automobile crashes, recreational accidents, on-the-job accidents, and death by homicide and suicide. Moreover, U.S. alcoholism and alcohol abuse cost society approximately $200 billion per year. In human terms, the costs are incalculable for those who have suffered personally, psychologically, physically, and economically. Some statistics are summarized in Box 1.2: Harmful Effects of Alcoholism and Alcohol Abuse.

BOX 1.2: Harmful Effects of Alcoholism and Alcohol Abuse

Effects on Health

- There are more than 2 million alcohol-related deaths worldwide each year.

- Alcohol abuse is responsible for more than 60 types of disease and injury. The WHO estimates that 20% to 30% of esophageal cancers, liver cancers, and cirrhosis of the liver, homicides, epilepsy, and motor vehicle accidents are alcohol related. Alcoholism is also a risk factor for one of the top killers worldwide: cardiovascular disease. (www.america.gov/st/health-english/2008/October/2008 1023115119abretnuh0.9323999.html)

General United States Drunk Driving Statistics

- Alcohol-related car crashes kill someone every 45 minutes and injure someone every 2 minutes.

- In the United States, drunk driving is the leading criminal cause of death.

- More than 17,000 people are the victims of drunk driving accidents every year.

- Approximately 40% of all motor-vehicle fatalities are alcohol related.

- Frequent drunk drivers are responsible for almost 60% of alcohol-related fatalities.

BOX 1.2 *Continued*

- 38% of all Christmas-time car accident deaths and 54% of all New Year car accident deaths are alcohol related.

- Approximately 17% of drunk drivers injured in car accidents are charged and convicted, 11% are charged and not convicted, and 72% are never charged.

- Drunk driving accidents cost the public around $200 billion a year.

- About one third of people arrested for drunk driving are repeat offenders.

- Drivers with a blood alcohol levels of .08 or higher who are involved in fatal crashes are eight times more likely to have a prior DUI conviction than drivers who consumed no alcohol. (www.edgarsnyder.com/drunk-driving/statistics.html)

- 1,347 children ages 14 and younger died as occupants in car accidents in 2008. Of those deaths, 216 (approx 16%) were the direct result of drunk drivers.

- Along with the 1,347 child occupant fatalities, another 34 children died as pedestrians or bikers who were hit by drunk drivers. (http://www.america. gov/st/health-english/2008/October/20081023115119abretnuh0.9323999. html#ixzz0fR6MS8tn)

Assault Statistics and Alcoholism

- Two thirds of victims of intimate partner violence were connected with alcohol use or abuse. (www.ojp.usdoj.gov/bjs/pub/pdf/ac.pdf)

- More than 70,000 students between the ages of 18 and 24 were victims of alcohol-related sexual assault in the U.S.

- An estimated 480,000 children are mistreated each year by a caretaker with alcohol problems. (Children of Alcoholics Foundation, 1996)

- Communities and neighborhoods that have more bars and liquor stores per capita experience more assaults. (Scribner, MacKinnon & Dwyer, 1995)

BOX 1.2 *Continued*

- 30% of the most severe incidents involving men as victims, from both the general population and college samples, occurred in or around a bar. (Quigley, Leonard, & Collins, 2003)

- Excessive alcohol use causes an estimated 79,000 deaths per year in the United States. Unlike other drugs, alcohol disperses in all body tissues and therefore has the potential to harm many organ systems such as cancer of the liver, head, neck, esophagus, and female breast. (Alcohol-Attributable Deaths Report, Average for United States 2001–2005, National Center for Chronic Disease Prevention and Health Promotion, Centers for Disease Control and Prevention)

- Chronic heavy drinking is a leading cause of cardiovascular disease.

- Long-term alcohol abuse destroys the cerebellum, the brain region responsible for sensory perception, coordination, and motor control.

- Alcohol dependence and abuse cost the US approximately $220 billion in 2005. For the sake of comparison, this was greater than the amount of money spent to combat cancer ($196 billion) and obesity ($133 billion). (www.america.gov/st/health-english/2008/October/20081023115119abretnuh0.9323999.html)

- In 2006, more than 19% of drivers aged 16 to 20 who died in motor vehicle crashes had been drinking alcohol. (National Highway Traffic Safety Administration; Traffic Safety Facts 2006: Alcohol-Impaired Driving; www.nrd.nhtsa.dot.gov/Pubs/810801.PDF)

Strategies and Interventions

Just as there has been much discussion, research, and follow-up with the various issues, there has also been an array of procedures, strategies, programs, and structured organizations designed to ameliorate the problem and support alcoholics themselves. These support services differ on the basis of their analysis of the problem and in the nature of the interventions provided. For example, there are medical services that are hospital or clinically based which provide detoxification and follow-up programs. Other programs, such as Alcoholics Anonymous, place strong emphasis on group support, mentoring and sponsorship where the individual is provided with direction and support for life. In addition, there are many self-help programs which are based on the individual's capacity and willingness to follow a plan with on-going self-assessment, checklists, and strategies. Specific details on these approaches will be incorporated into the latter sections of this book where strategies for each phase of alcoholism are addressed.

Regulation of Alcohol Use

In addition to the array of support services available to alcoholics, there has been a significant increase in regulation of the use, availability, and access to alcohol. For example, the state liquor control commissions and licensing agencies have increased monitoring of alcohol use and distribution, serving of alcohol to minors, and of patrons who may be intoxicated. The police have become increasingly active in monitoring drivers who may be under the influence, particularly at critical drinking times such as the New Year period, national holidays, and special events. Also the courts have increased fines and penalties for driving under the influence of alcohol.

These efforts have resulted in some limited success in curbing or containing excessive alcohol use and its harmful effects, especially on reducing road fatalities and accidents (http://pubs.niaaa.nih.gov/publications/arh25-1/32-42.htm; http://copsandcourts.com/?p=960).

Trends

Given there has been on-going research on issues related to alcoholism, continued availability of an array of support services, greater controls exerted by state liquor control commissions, and increasing accountability and activity through the courts, two questions arise: Has the incidence of alcohol abuse been reduced? What are the trends regarding excessive alcohol consumption?

The Department of Health and Human Services, Centers of Disease Control and Prevention (www.cdc.gov) conduct surveys on various aspects of health and diseases at a national level on an annual basis. One particular national survey addressed the trends in alcohol consumption over the period 1993–2007. Respondents were categorized into two groups first: binge drinking was defined as respondents who reported five or more drinks on an occasion. The second group, heavy drinking was defined as respondents who reported an average of two or more drinks per day (www.cdc.gov/alcohol/datatable.htm). The trend for both groups showed a steady increase in drinking from 1993 to 2002, a slight change in 2003, followed by a reduction in consumption for the period 2004 to 2007. The overall trend from 1993 to 2007 showed an increase of approximately 22% for binge drinking (14.2 million to 15.8 million) and an increase of approximately 73% for heavy drinking (3.0 million to 5.2 million). These results are depicted in Table 1.1. Based on these data, the conclusion is that alcohol consumption over this 15-year period has shown an *overall increase* in the United States.

TABLE 1.1: Prevalence of Binge Drinking and Heavy Drinking among Adults in U.S. 1993–2007											
	1993	1995	1997	1999	2001	2002	2003	2004	2005	2006	2007
Binge Drinking (in millions)	14.2	14.1	14.5	14.9	14.8	16.3	16.5	15.1	14.4	15.4	15.8
HeavyDrinking (in millions)	3.0	2.9	3.0	3.7	5.1	5.9	5.8	4.9	4.9	4.9	5.2

Source: www.cdc.gov/alcohol/datatable.htm

July 30, 2010 Gallup Poll (www.gallup.com.) reported that 67% of U.S. adults drink alcohol, which represents a slight increase over the previous year. However, the percentage of Americans who report drinking alcohol has been relatively stable over the 71 years that Gallup has been tracking this trend.

The reader may pursue some of these topics in more depth by referring to the following additional resources listed in Box 1.3.

BOX 1.3: Additional Resources on Background Information on Alcoholism

Alcoholics Anonymous, 4th Edition, (2001). New York, NY: Alcoholics Anonymous World Services.

Jellinek, E. M., (1960). *The Disease Concept of Alcoholism*. New Haven, CT: Hillhouse.

Ketcham, K., Asbury, W. F., Schulstad, M., & Ciaramicoli, A. P. (2000). *Beyond the Influence: Understanding and Defeating Alcoholism*. New York: Bantam Books.

Martinic, M., & Leigh, B. (2004). *Reasonable Risk-Alcohol in Perspective*. New York: Brunner-Routledge.

Oltmanns, T. F. & Emery, R. E. (2010). *Abnormal Psychology* (6th ed.). Upper Saddle River, NJ: Prentice Hall.

Chapter Summary

Excessive use of alcohol is a long-standing national and worldwide problem. The deleterious effects of alcoholism have been felt in every corner of our culture from children to adults, among individuals, friends and families, and in all walks of life. Everyone knows someone who is struggling with this problem.

There has been much discussion, writing, and research on defining and formulating various levels or categories of alcohol use. The etiologies of alcoholism and risk factors have been well documented. The harmful effects of excessive drinking of alcohol are staggering and all too familiar. An array of support services for alcoholics is relatively easy to access. In addition, government agencies and the courts have become increasingly active in regulating the use of alcohol and establishing serious consequences for behavior related to excessive drinking.

Given the scope and intensity of these efforts at all levels, we might expect that the problems of alcoholism are coming under control. There are certainly indicators that problems have been curbed in that the harmful effects have been reduced. There is the undeniable fact, however, that alcohol consumption has shown *a steady increase over recent decades*. This trend clearly implies that all the risks associated with alcoholism are still prevalent.

Whereas there is no claim that this book will solve these problems, the need still exists for workable and effective approaches and strategies for helping individuals understand and address the problem of alcoholism. This book provides tools to meet this need and describes skills for establishing healthy sobriety.

Understanding the Pathway to Alcoholism

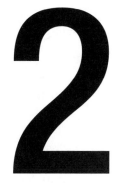

We forge the chains we wear in life.

— Charles Dickens

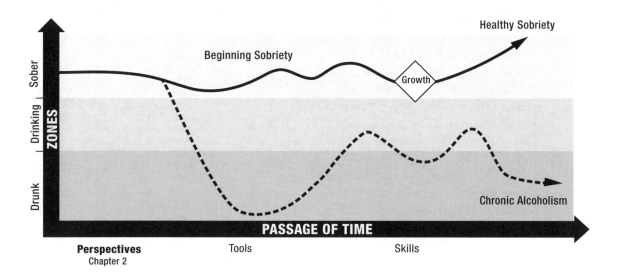

Alcoholism is an incredibly pervasive and far-reaching problem that significantly affects people of all ages, walks of life, gender, ethnic groups, and geographical locations. Given this extraordinary range of influence and effect, it might seem an ambitious or possibly naïve undertaking to construct a model that helps to understand why people begin drinking in the first place and then become addicted. Or, it might be concluded that there is indeed a challenge to sift through the volumes of information and listen to the myriad of personal stories to distill patterns and explanations. The purpose of this book is to describe the process in which alcoholism is established and to present a model for depicting the pathway to alcoholism. Once this pathway is understood, tools will provided for alcoholics and support personnel to develop an alternative pathway for lifelong recovery from alcoholism.

The following model arose from several sources: the first authors' research and practice with this model addressing serious problem behavior in other fields; extensive reading on the subject of alcoholism; work in the field; and in interviewing many individuals who considered themselves to be recovering alcoholics. The kinds of questions that were investigated are listed in Box 2.1: Interview Questions for Alcoholics.

BOX 2.1: Interview Questions for Alcoholics

Why did you start drinking in the first place?

What circumstances led you to drink?

What were the triggers for drinking?

What do you think you got from drinking?

What were the positive effects from drinking?

What were the negative or harmful effects from drinking?

Were there any changes in how often you turned to alcohol?

Were there any changes in how much you consumed?

Were there changes in your reasons for drinking?

Have you tried to quit drinking?

What did you do to quit?

If you were successful in quitting, what do you attribute the success to?

What do you do to stay sober?

Responses to these questions began to show a fairly clear pattern. Individuals would begin to use alcohol to address certain needs they have. For example, individuals may experience loneliness in the evening, so they gravitate to a bar to gather with others for a drink rather than stay home alone. These kinds of social events were not part of the individual's present life so drinking alcohol at gatherings like this *met a real need* for the person. Consequently, whenever this person felt the need for company he or she could head to a bar and have some drinks. The need would be met. Some individuals would develop a pattern of heading to the bar at certain times of the day or weekend to visit with others, and to have a few drinks on a regular basis.

In some cases, however, the individual would begin to stay longer at the bars or go there more frequently to meet their social needs, and it is not that long before the individual just had to go to the bar for the *alcohol*. In other words the consumption of alcohol becomes the *primary* need for going to the bar and the need for companionship becomes secondary. Once the need to drink becomes firmly established, the stage for alcoholism is set.

In this chapter behavioral analyses is described which shows how alcoholism is established in the first place and secondly how it is maintained. This model is used to help understand the cycle of alcohol use leading to alcoholism and the implications for addressing alcoholism in the design of recovery plans. Topics addressed are: 1. The basics of a behavioral model, 2. Establishing behavior cycles, 3. Application of the behavior cycle model to alcohol use, 4. The shift from alcohol use to alcohol dependence, 5. A model for the pathway to alcoholism, and 6. Implications for recovery tools.

The Basics of a Behavioral Model

The most basic form of a behavioral model used to explain how behavior cycles are established consists of three parts, a. triggers, b. responses, and c. effects.

Triggers

Triggers refer to the events, needs, or circumstances that set the stage for a person to act. Triggers have also been called stimuli, antecedents, needs, circumstances, situations, conditions, dispositions or feelings, contexts, and events. Here are some examples of triggers:

- A person may feel hungry. The feeling of hunger is the trigger that sets the occasion for the person to eat.

- A person may experience loneliness and want to be with others. The feeling of loneliness is the trigger that prompts the person to get with others.

> **Triggers** are those factors that set the occasion for a person to take action.

- An individual may feel stress from an intolerable employment situation. The stress is the trigger that may encourage the person to skip work.

- A customer wants a drink at a bar and is trying to get the bartender's attention. The trigger is wanting a drink and inability to get the bartender's attention. The customer may then call out to the bartender requesting a drink.

- The individual may want to celebrate a special occasion. The trigger is the need to celebrate an event.

Responses

Responses are the actions an individual takes to address the triggers. Responses have also been referred to as behaviors, actions, or specific responses such as fighting, running away, drinking alcohol, or visiting a friend. Typically the individual chooses actions that specifically address the triggers currently being experienced. From the five examples above under the heading Triggers, the respective triggers and possible corresponding responses are listed in Box 2.2: Examples of Triggers and Responses in the Behavioral Model.

> **Responses** are those actions taken by an individual in the presence of certain triggers.

BOX 2.2: Examples of Triggers and Responses in the Behavioral Model	
Triggers	**Responses**
Person feels hungry	Eats something
Experiences loneliness	Gets together with others
Feels stress from work	Skips some work days
Wants a drink at the bar	Calls out to bartender
Desires to celebrate an event	Organizes a party

Effects

Effects refer to the results of the actions taken by an individual. Other names used for effects include consequences, repercussions, results, impacts, outcomes, and functions. A cornerstone of the behavioral model is to fully understand the way the *effects* work for the individual. These effects, in the traditional behavioral model, have been described in terms of reinforcement theory in which two types of reinforcement can occur. First, the individual gets something that is desirable through a particular behavior that is called *positive reinforcement.* Second, the individual may be successful in removing something that is undesirable through a behavior which is called *negative reinforcement.* Each of these possibilities, positive and negative reinforcement, is operative in the development and maintenance of alcoholism. For example, the response of the person who calls out in a bar has the effect of getting the bartender's attention and then a drink. By calling out, the individual gets something desired (in this case a drink). The behavior of calling out in the bar has been *positively reinforced.*

> **Effects** are the results of a response in which the individual may get something needed (positive reinforcement), or remove something undesirable (negative reinforcement).

In another example, the person who is having a hard time at work skips a few days and by doing so is effective in removing something he does not like (specifically a tough time at work). In this case the behavior of skipping a few days of work has been *negatively reinforced*.

Sometimes there is confusion between punishment and negative reinforcement. Punishment is designed to *reduce a behavior* by presenting something negative. For example, an individual is fined (something negative) for speeding. The idea is that the behavior of speeding will be reduced through the negative consequence of a fine. Negative reinforcement, on the other hand, is designed to *increase a behavior* by removing or reducing something that is negative. For example, a person's insurance is reduced (reducing something negative) for a good driving record. By reducing the insurance premium, good driving is likely to be increased.

The possible effects of the responses to the triggers identified in the examples in Box 2.2 are listed in Box 2.3: Examples of Effects of Responses to Triggers.

BOX 2.3: Examples of Effects of Responses to Triggers		
Triggers	**Responses**	**Effects (Reinforcement)**
Person feels hungry	Eats something	No longer hungry (removes something undesirable– negative reinforcement)
Experiences loneliness	Gets together with others	No longer lonely (removes something undesirable– negative reinforcement)
Feels stress from work	Skips some work days	Settles down some (removes something undesirable– negative reinforcement)
Wants a drink at the bar	Calls bartender for a drink	Drink is delivered (gets something– positive reinforcement)
Desire to celebrate an event	Organizes a party	Has fun with friends (gets something– positive reinforcement)

Establishing Behavior Cycles

Behavior cycles describe the process in which an individual is very likely to make the same response in the presence of future occurrences of certain triggers because *it works*—it is reinforced. That is, the *effects* of the responses enable the individual to get what is desired (positive reinforcement) or remove something that is undesirable (negative reinforcement). This means that if the same, or similar triggers arise in the future, the individual is likely to make the same response again. The logic is that the response worked before, so it is likely to work again. Naturally, if the response has the same effect, the individual will keep making this response under these conditions. In other words, the response *is now established* and a cycle of responding in this way will continue.

This cyclical relationship between the three components in a behavioral model of *triggers, responses*, and *effects* is depicted in Figure 2.1: Establishing a Behavior Cycle. The arrows show the links between the components of the model, specifically triggers lead to responses that are then reinforced. This pathway continues with future occurrences of the presence of the same or similar triggers leading to an habitual behavior cycle.

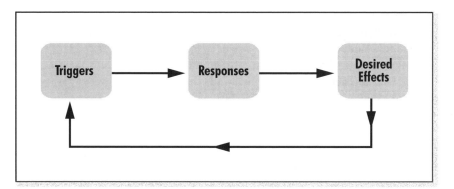

FIGURE 2.1: Establishing a Behavior Cycle

More in-depth information on the behavioral model and its components are listed in Box 2.4: Additional Resources on the Behavioral Model.

BOX 2.4: Additional Resources on the Behavioral Model

Carr, J., & Wilder, D. A. (2004). *Functional Assessment and Intervention: A Guide to Understanding Behavior* (2nd ed.). Homewood, IL: High Tide Press.

Colvin, G. (2004). *Managing the Cycle of Acting-Out Behavior in the Classroom.* Eugene, OR: Behavior Associates.

Colvin, G. (2009). *Managing Noncompliance and Defiance in the Classroom: A Road Map for Teachers, Specialists, and Behavior Support Teams.* Thousand Oaks, CA: Corwin.

Cooper, J. O., Heron, T. E., & Heward, W. L. (2007). *Applied Behavior Analysis* (2nd ed.). Upper Saddle River, NJ: Pearson Education.

Application of the Behavior Cycle Model to Alcohol Use

One way of trying to understand the complexity of alcohol use and alcoholism is to apply alcohol use to the behavior cycle model. In this model the *triggers* component becomes any perceived *need* that arises for an individual, and the *response* component becomes alcohol use which give rise to *effects* that meet this need (either getting something desirable or removing something undesirable). By using alcohol in the presence of certain needs, the individual finds that these needs are met as a result of consuming alcohol. Here are three illustrations.

> **Illustration 1.** Bill has been having rough days at work and comes home experiencing a lot of stress. He finds it hard to relax at home and has trouble getting to sleep. A friend suggested he have a couple of glasses of wine in the evening, which he did. He found that he relaxed, forgot about work problems, and, for the first time in a while, he had a good night's sleep. Thereafter, each evening he would have a couple of glasses of wine to settle down and to sleep.

In this scenario, the *triggers* were stress from work and the need was to obtain relief from that stress. In addition he needed sleep. The *response* was to take a couple of glasses of wine; and the *effects* were a reduction in stress, settling down, forgetting about work, and having a good night's sleep. Drinking alcohol was negatively reinforced because the stress was reduced (something undesired was removed) and was also positively reinforced because sleep (something desired) was achieved.

> **Illustration 2.** Joanne had just received a significant promotion at work and there was a small party at the office with cake and soft drinks to celebrate the event. While Joanne appreciated her coworkers gathering to acknowledge her promotion, she still felt the need to celebrate and feel the joy of her accomplishment. The office party seemed a little stilted and formal. So, after work, she invited a few friends to her house to celebrate and have a few drinks. It was not long before there was much laughter, approval, exchanges of hugs, storytelling, and singing. When her friends left she felt somewhat giddy, happy, and satisfied.

In this illustration the *triggers* for Joanne were the need to celebrate and feel happy and satisfied. The *response* was to arrange a party at her home with friends and the *effects* were much enjoyment, approval and positive interactions.

> **Illustration 3.** Sarah always found she was intimidated in a group situation where others would be talking and she would be expected to participate. She found she would choke up or be quite fearful of saying something that might be considered stupid. One afternoon she was sitting with a group at a friend's home and had the usual feelings of intimidation and inhibition. The friend brought out some beer, wine, and soft drinks and surprisingly offered her a beer, which she accepted. She found sipping the beer gave her something to do while the group was chatting. After she had a few beers, she found she was very relaxed and surprised herself by recounting an incident from work. She was also gratified that others showed considerable interest in her story. Sarah made the connection that the alcohol loosened her up, helped her to be less intimidated, and removed the inhibitions of talking in the group. She then began to seek out gatherings where alcohol was available and had the same experience each time, namely that the alcohol helped her participate more fully and more freely in the group.

In this example, for Sarah the *triggers, unmet needs,* were feelings of intimidation and inhibition in a group; the *response* was to drink beer; and the *effects* were a reduction in intimidation and inhibition enabling her to talk more freely in the group and gain more acceptance from the group.

The use of alcohol in a behavior cycle for each of these three examples, Bill, Joanne, and Sarah, are summarized in Box 2.5: Illustrations of Behavior Cycle with Alcohol Use.

BOX 2.5: Illustrations of Behavior Cycle with Alcohol Use			
	Triggers	**Responses**	**Effects**
Illustration #1 Bill	Comes home stressed from work, cannot relax, has trouble sleeping	Drinks a couple of glasses of wine at home	Begins to relax (negative reinforcement) Is able to sleep (positive reinforcement)
Illustration #2 Joanne	Wants to celebrate, feel happy and satisfied	Has party at home with alcohol	Much enjoyment: laughter, approval, hugs, stories, and singing (positive reinforcement)
Illustration ##3 Sarah	Feels intimidated and inhibited in a group	Has a few beers	Feels less intimidated Loses inhibitions (negative reinforcement) Contributes and experiences acceptance from group (positive reinforcement)

Critical Note: It is particularly important to understand that the effects induced by alcohol are *relatively swift*. For example, in the illustrations above, after just a few drinks Bill was feeling quite relaxed. Similarly, Sarah found that she became more confident quite quickly after just a couple of drinks. Consequently, it is predictable that certain individuals will continue to use alcohol to reduce stress, deal with lack of confidence, and meet other needs even though the relief is short term. However, these short-term benefits make it worthwhile to pursue the use of alcohol for these individuals when everything else that has been tried has not worked for them. For this reason alcohol *is a powerful reinforcer* (albeit a short-term remedy).

In general, alcohol use, how it can be established as a routine or habit, can be described in terms of a behavior cycle. This cyclical relationship between the three components in a behavioral model of *triggers, responses,* and *effects* applies to alcohol use and abuse where the triggers component is typically a *need,* the response component is *alcohol use,* and the effects are *positive and negative reinforcement* where the individual gets something desirable and/or removes something undesirable. This model is depicted in Figure 2.2: Establishing a Behavior Cycle of Alcohol Use.

Summary Point

Alcohol has an important unique property of being able to meet people's needs VERY QUICKLY which is a major reason why some people return to drinking alcohol so readily.

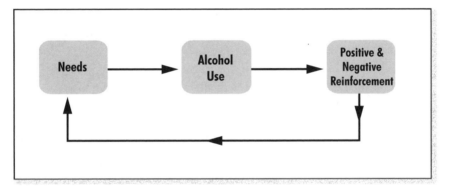

FIGURE 2.2: Establishing a Behavior Cycle of Alcohol Use

In Section Two when tools are introduced for recovery, it will be critical for the reader to clearly identify the specific details of the *triggers*/unmet needs, *the responses*/use of alcohol, and the *effects*/reinforcement for an alcoholic. Guidelines and checklists will be provided in Section Two to assist the reader with pinpointing these details.

The Shift from Alcohol Use to Alcohol Dependence

At this juncture we have described the use of alcohol in terms of a behavioral model where certain needs are met by consuming alcohol. Once the person begins to consume alcohol, effects come into play which meet these needs by providing something desirable (positive reinforcement) and/or by removing something undesirable (negative reinforcement). When the same needs arise in the future, the person will often turn to alcohol to meet the needs. The use of alcohol under these conditions then becomes a regular practice. Many people are able to restrict their drinking to these occasions and control how much they drink. This situation is very common and can be considered the norm for many people in society. However, this is not the case for everyone. This is not the case for the alcoholic.

One of the most challenging aspects in addressing the problem of alcoholism is to understand when and why an individual shifts from being one who *uses alcohol* to one who *abuses alcohol* and becomes an *alcoholic*. There is a shift from drinking alcohol under certain conditions that the individual can control, to one where the alcohol controls the individual. This shift occurs when a person's use of alcohol begins in a limited way for quite specific reasons then, over time, the use of alcohol becomes more controlling and its use is extended to other times and needs. As F. Scott Fitzgerald so aptly said :

> "First you take a drink, then the drink takes a drink, then the drink takes you."

The person begins to look for alcohol at any time—or under any circumstance. Some individuals, in effect, develop an *all-consuming* and *irresistible need* for alcohol. They become dependent on alcohol. They become alcoholics.

The key to understanding the transition from regular alcohol use to alcoholism lies in the changing nature of the needs and effects. The *needs* now become *cravings*. Initially, an individual turns to alcohol to meet a certain need. For example, the person may go to a bar for company, someone to talk to, and drink some alcohol. The alcohol gives access to company which meets the person's need. However, when the person finds more occasions to drink and consumes more alcohol on these occasions, t*he effects of alcohol itself* take over from the initial effects (such as needing company). The effects of alcohol on the individual become the primary purpose for drinking while the initial needs (e.g., company)

Alcohol cravings are best described as intense physical, mental, and emotional urges to drink alcohol. The direct effect of alcohol becomes the primary reason for drinking.

become secondary or irrelevant. A cycle begins to develop between the needs, now cravings, and the powerful effects of alcohol.

While it may be difficult to fully understand the physiological mechanisms and processes for when a person shifts from being a controlled alcohol user to an uncontrolled alcoholic—several salient particulars are noted in Box 2.6: Particulars in the Transition from Alcohol Use to Alcoholism.

BOX 2.6: Particulars in the Transition from Alcohol Use to Alcoholism

- The individual develops a craving for alcohol that is an irresistible and overpowering urge to drink.

- The cravings now become physical with the person having the shakes, headaches, and other physical symptoms that are not relieved until alcohol is consumed.

- Individuals can also experience strong mental and emotional triggers such as intense anxiety, panic, restlessness, agitation, and anguish until they have consumed alcohol.

- The craving for alcohol is not really satisfied as the alcoholic continues to drink until collapsing or staggering off to sleep. It is as if the "thirst" cannot be quenched.

- The cravings become so strong that even severe repercussions, such as weakening or destruction of relationships or putting a job in jeopardy, do not make any difference.

- The individual begins to use alcohol at additional times and places to meet other needs. The person begins to drink more frequently and consume more at these additional times and places. In effect, more triggers come into play.

- The switch from regular alcohol use to alcohol abuse can occur over a very wide range of time from two years up to sixty years.

- Typically alcoholics cannot revert to regular alcohol use. The vast majority of alcoholics who quit drinking and start up again become alcoholics again. This process of reversion is called a relapse

- Those who begin with alcohol abuse and have alcoholism in their family history are likely to become alcoholics.

- The effects of alcohol become the triggers, now cravings. Once the person gets the "buzz" from drinking, drinking must continue to maintain or increase this buzz.

For the person experiencing these cravings, relief is only obtained by drinking alcohol. The cravings can occur at any time of the day and will not be quelled or mollified until alcohol is consumed. Moreover, the cravings are only reduced for a short time then the urges to drink start up again and again. The diagram in Figure 2.3 shows the transition from alcohol use to alcoholism where the triggers become cravings and the effects of drinking alcohol become directly linked to the cravings.

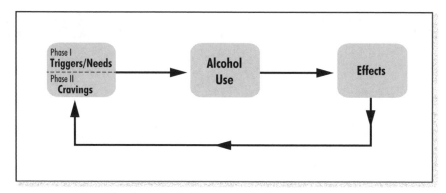

FIGURE 2.3: Transition from Alcohol Use to Alcoholism

More in-depth information on this subject of the causes, mechanisms, and process for the transition of alcohol use to alcoholism are cited in Box 2.7: Additional Resources on Transition from Alcohol Use to Alcoholism.

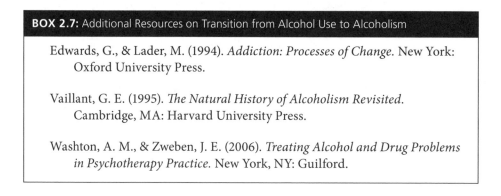

BOX 2.7: Additional Resources on Transition from Alcohol Use to Alcoholism

Edwards, G., & Lader, M. (1994). *Addiction: Processes of Change.* New York: Oxford University Press.

Vaillant, G. E. (1995). *The Natural History of Alcoholism Revisited.* Cambridge, MA: Harvard University Press.

Washton, A. M., & Zweben, J. E. (2006). *Treating Alcohol and Drug Problems in Psychotherapy Practice.* New York, NY: Guilford.

A Model for the Pathway to Alcoholism

The behavior of a person who has become dependent on alcohol, has progressed from social or controlled drinking to uncontrolled drinking, follows a fairly predictable pattern. This pattern can be depicted as a model, described as a *pathway to alcoholism*. The model is presented in terms of 1. A behavior escalation cycle in seven phases, and 2. Description of pathway to alcoholism.

A Behavior Escalation Cycle in Seven Phases

The first author developed a widely used and extensively published model for educators and service providers to use in public schools and institutions for managing serious acting-out behavior (Colvin, 2010; Colvin, 2004; Colvin 1999). These acting-out behaviors include severe tantrums, serious disruptive behavior, explosive behavior, emotional escalation, violence, meltdowns, aggression, and self-abuse which, as expected, pose significant challenges to educators. Colvin described these behaviors in terms of an escalation cycle composed of seven phases:

1. **Calm** where the individual is basically on track with the class activity.

2. **Triggers** come into play that set off the individual.

3. **Agitation** is the phase reached once the triggers begin to operate and the individual becomes upset.

4. **Acceleration** is when the individual's behavior begins to worsen.

5. **Peak** is the phase where the individual is out of control and the serious behavior occurs.

6. **De-escalation** is the period following a serious phase 5 incident where the individual begins to settle down and recover.

7. **Recovery** is where the individual has regained control of himself or herself and resumes the class activity.

While this sequence is briefly described as a single incident, this is usually not the case. Once the triggers reappear, the individual is very likely to follow the same pathway of reaching serious acting-out behavior, de-escalating, back to the recovery phase, and starting over again. This cycle of acting-out behavior is represented in Figure 2.4. (Colvin, 2004).

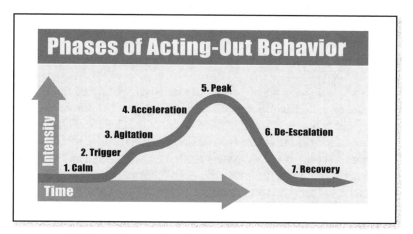

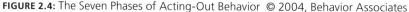

FIGURE 2.4: The Seven Phases of Acting-Out Behavior © 2004, Behavior Associates

The utility of this model lies in pinpointing where interventions can and need to be made. Strategies are generated for each phase in this model. Consequently, once individuals display where they are in the cycle, educators and service providers can implement interventions directly which, ideally, will interrupt the cycle at this point so that no further escalation will occur. Emphasis in this model is placed on intervening as *early as possible* in the cycle so that subsequent problem behavior is prevented. More in-depth resources are listed in Box 2.8.

BOX 2.8: Resources for Addressing Serious Acting-Out Behavior in Schools & Institutions

Colvin, G. (1999). *Defusing Anger and Aggression: Safe Strategies for Secondary School Educators* [Video/DVD program]. Eugene, OR: Iris Media.

Colvin, G. (2004). *Managing the Cycle of Acting-out Behavior in the Classroom*. Eugene, OR: Behavior Associates.

Colvin, G. (2009). *Managing the Cycle of Emotional Escalation*. In R. Sprick & M. Garrison (Eds.), Interventions: Evidence-Based Behavioral Strategies of Individual Students (2nd ed., pp. 425–462). Eugene, OR: Pacific Northwest Publishing.

Colvin, G. (2010). *Defusing Disruptive Behavior in the Classroom*. Thousand Oaks, CA: Corwin.

Colvin, G., & Sheehan, M. (2012). *Managing the Cycle of Meltdowns for Students with Autism Spectrum Disorder*. Thousand Oaks, CA: Corwin.

Beginning Pathway to Alcoholism

This model for acting-out behavior has direct application for describing the cycle of alcoholism and has clear implications for interventions. Alcoholism can be depicted as a series of identifiable phases similar to the seven-phase series described for acting-out behavior by students in schools. The individual starts out sober, triggers and cravings come into play, the individual begins drinking and continues until a drunken state is reached resulting in on-going serious repercussions. A *moment of clarity* often occurs, drinking ceases temporarily, and the cycle begins again. This series of phases is called a *pathway to alcoholism*. A model for this pathway is presented in Figure 2.5: Pathway to Beginning Alcoholism. The vertical axis, called *Zones*, is divided into three parts, *Sober, Drinking,* and *Drunk*. The horizontal axis called a *Passage of Time,* shows that changes occur over time. The graph depicts the various phases, 1 through 7, the terms of which are described below.

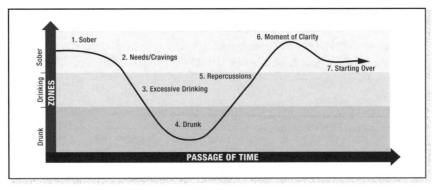

FIGURE 2.5: Pathway to Beginning Alcoholism

Descriptions of Pathway Terms

1. **Sober** in this book means alcohol free. If a person has not had an alcoholic drink for three days, then that person has been sober for three days. The legal definition of sober is simply a measure of percentage blood alcohol levels, usually below 0.5%. As long as the person is under the mandated level, then he or she is considered to be sober by law. However, for the purpose of developing an alternative healthier pathway to alcoholism, the goal of this book, sober is used in the sense of *zero intake of alcohol.*

2. **Needs/Cravings** have been linked because, as described earlier in this chapter, triggers give way to cravings—there is a progression between triggers and cravings. A person begins to drink because of certain needs that are not met, called triggers. These needs are often stress related such as loss of job, long days at work, and conflicts in relationships. Other triggers are personal and social needs such as lack of confidence or feeling lonely. Drinking alcohol serves as short-term relief from these triggers. The person after consuming alcohol starts to relax, enjoy other people's company, and gains some confidence.

    However, in many cases, the needs progress to cravings. That is the person begins to yearn for alcohol in itself and for itself. The person begins to drink for the effects alcohol has on the mind and body. The body itself begins to urgently desire alcohol. This desire is analogous to pangs of hunger where the stomach growls for food after sustained deprivation. Cravings manifest themselves as having the shakes, the fixation on the need to drink, and the loss of awareness or interest in anything else that might be happening at the moment. Basically, the person is consumed by the need to drink.

3. **Excessive Drinking** is inevitable for alcoholics once they begin to drink. Alcoholics, by definition, have little or no control over their drinking. Nonalcoholics, by contrast, can drink to their limit and quit. Once alcoholics begin to drink, excessive drinking becomes the norm. They cannot stop.

4. **Drunk** is clearly the stage reached once a person engages in excessive drinking. Drunkenness is usually expressed in the form of loss of physical control and coordination, slurred and broken speech, anger outbursts, inappropriate physical and sexual advances toward others, physical reactions such as drooling and vomiting, and slurred incoherent and repetitive speech. Drunken individuals may display loss of inhibitions or social skills by stripping off their clothes, climbing on tables, shouting, and singing. Overall, the individuals lose control of themselves physically, emotionally, and mentally.

5. **Repercussions** refer to the consequences or effects of being drunk or from being drunk frequently. The outcomes can be related to family scenes; police intervention from driving under the influence or drunk and disorderly conduct; hangovers and sickness the following day (or later that day); irregularities at work such as being late or being dysfunctional; significantly impaired judgment; injuries from fighting; victim of assault or theft; vehicular accident; and long-term damage to vital organs—the heart, liver, and kidneys. Alcoholics often report that they cannot remember events or incidents that occurred while they were drunk. The list continues and overall results of becoming drunk on a regular basis are particularly damaging to self, others, family, and careers.

6. **Moment of Clarity.** This moment, sometimes called an "aha" moment, occurs, in most cases, when the person ceases drinking and becomes aware of the repercussions following the last bout of drinking. It may be the individual sees very clearly the effects drinking have on self, own career, or health, and on others. This moment may come suddenly through what someone says; through sitting and thinking (perhaps in jail); the look on someone's face; a visual of an incident; or a close look at a car that was damaged from driving drunk. In effect, the individual has a sudden realization that big changes

need to occur. In addition, a moment of clarity need not be something sensational or horrific. Rather, some moments may be related to quite ordinary events but seen with a new perspective.

Note: This portion of the graph takes a little dip in the pathway to beginning alcoholism following the repercussion's phase and then begins to swing upwards. The reason for this is that the individual is thinking very clearly but it is transitory, hence the term "moment of clarity."

7. **Starting Over** occurs when the individual has regained some level of sobriety and is rested following a night's sleep (or rest from passing out). At this juncture the person has the opportunity of taking steps toward recovery and dealing with alcoholism or continuing the same pathway leading to excessive drinking, drunkenness, repercussions, and starting over the next day. This book is designed to help the alcoholic develop a competing pathway toward lifelong recovery rather than the pathway to alcoholism.

Established Pathway to Alcoholism

In many cases, individuals begin with the pathway to alcoholism and experience the cycle as follows: being sober→ using alcohol to meet certain needs→ drinking to reduce cravings→ becoming drunk→ becoming sober→ having moments of clarity→ and starting the cycle over again (see Figure 2.5: Pathway to Beginning Alcoholism). However, some of these individuals once they complete the cycle a few times become chronic alcoholics. That is, they do not return to a sober state. They remain either drunk, hung over, feeling the repercussions of excessive drinking, and resume as soon as they can. Now alcoholism has been established. In Figure 2.6, Pathway to Chronic Alcoholism, the solid line on the graph shows the individual remaining in the drinking/drunk zones. This established pathway has now replaced the beginning pathway to alcoholism (broken line on the graph).

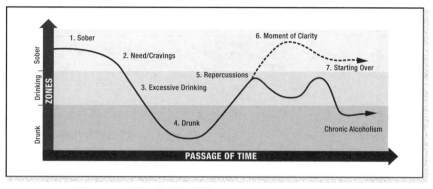

FIGURE 2.6: Pathway to Chronic Alcoholism

Implications for Recovery Tools

Understanding this concept of a *pathway to alcoholism* depicted in Figures 2.5 and 2.6 is central to this book. The three beginning phases of *sober, unmet needs/ cravings,* and *excessive drinking* are the key target intervention areas for addressing alcoholism. The fundamental assumption is that alcoholism has been established through a cyclical pathway. In order for alcoholism to be brought under control, the individual has to establish an *alternative pathway* that leads to sobriety. For example, when unmet needs or cravings arise, instead of following the pathway of excessive drinking leading to drunkenness, the individual engages in other competing activities that meet the persons' needs in a constructive manner and thereby avert the pathway to alcoholism. In effect a *new pathway* is established. Figure 2.7: The Choices—Chronic Alcoholism or Healthy Sobriety, depicts this new pathway to sobriety which, ideally, replaces the pathway to alcoholism. However, significant interventions are needed to break up this established pathway to alcoholism. The remainder of this book, Chapters 4–13, provides descriptions of tools and skills needed to help alcoholics forge a new pathway to lifelong sobriety.

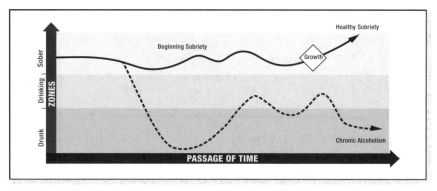

FIGURE 2.7: The Choices—Chronic Alcoholism or Healthy Sobriety

Chapter Summary

The use of alcohol has been, and still is, an integral part of society. Most people are capable of controlling how much they drink, when they drink, and their reasons for drinking. Some individuals, however, through continued use of alcohol, and no other effective strategies for meeting their needs, begin to expand its use and drink more. A transition occurs which brings about two changes. First, they shift from drinking for specific reasons, such as social needs, celebrations, or to experience relief, to drinking for the effect of alcohol itself. The initial reasons for drinking become quite secondary. Second, they begin to lose control over drinking, specifically, how much they drink and how often they drink. The triggers that set the occasion for alcohol use in a controlled way give way to cravings which lead to uncontrolled drinking.

A behavioral model was used to depict the processes for the transition from the cycle of alcohol use, to a establishing a pathway to alcoholism, and, alternatively, a pathway to sobriety. The behavioral model consists of three components: *triggers,* which are the needs a person may have; *responses*, the actions a person takes to meet these needs; and *effects*, which are the results or outcomes of the actions taken. If the effects meet the person's needs, then these responses will be repeated in the future when the same or similar triggers arise. This pattern was then depicted as a *pathway to alcoholism,* one of the cornerstones of this book. This pathway was divided into seven phases: sober, needs/cravings, excessive drinking, drunk, repercussions, moment of clarity, and starting over. For some individuals who follow this cycle a number of times, a pathway is established that stays within the drinking and drunk zones. Alcoholism has been established. The basic approach in this book is to use interventions to break up this pathway to alcoholism and to establish an alternative or competing pathway that leads to lifelong healthy sobriety. Tools and skills for establishing such a competing pathway are presented in the remaining sections of this book.

Making the Commitment

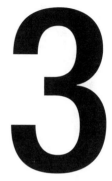

You must take personal responsibility. You cannot change the circumstances, the seasons, or the wind, but you can change yourself. That is something you have charge of.

– Jim Rohn

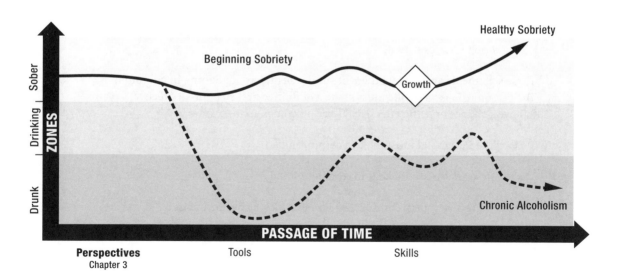

How often have statements like this been heard regarding the person who is an alcoholic?

- "Michael has so many likeable qualities, but he is an alcoholic and he will not do anything about his drinking."

- "Sarah has all the love one could ask for in her family, yet she will not take steps to stop drinking despite our pleadings."

- "Mario has been successful in his business and sports, but now that he is an alcoholic he won't accept that he can change. He seems to have given up."

- "If she would just take the first step and come to meetings or do something, but she won't."

- "We have offered to pay in full any costs associated with even residential treatment for Andy, but he just rolls his eyes and says that it is not time."

- "I don't know what it takes. She has lost her job, her children are mad at her, her husband is thinking of leaving her, yet she won't stop drinking."

- "I have arranged to pay a taxi to take Bert to meetings, church groups, or whatever he prefers, but he won't go."

- "Rhonda started a program at our urgings, but she quit after awhile. Her heart was never in it."

These statements and many others of similar bent, have one thing in common: The person who is alcoholic must make a definitive first step for any recovery plan to have a chance of being effective. Three outcomes are necessary:

1. The individual must make a commitment.

2. No one else can make it for the individual.

3. No recovery plan can succeed without such a commitment.

While the bulk of this section is devoted to details for effective recovery planning, this chapter addresses the challenging topic of *motivation*—the various elements involved in helping a person with alcoholism make the critical decision to quit drinking and embark on a recovery plan. The topics addressed are: 1. The nature of motivation; 2. Ten factors enabling alcoholics to make a commitment, and 3. Checklists and Action Plan.

The Nature of Motivation

Issues with motivation are not restricted to alcoholism. It seems that every organization has to wrestle aspects of motivation, such as how to get the most out of its members or how to get them to commit to being fully on board. Many examples come immediately to mind: the employer trying to coax employees to be more diligent and productive, the coach trying to motivate a super talented player who is not driven to succeed, the teacher trying to encourage students to elevate their achievement when they have settled for mediocrity, and parents frustrated with their children for not trying or not participating in activities when they have so much to offer.

In general, motivation can be divided into two main categories, extrinsic and intrinsic.

Extrinsic Motivation

As the name suggests, extrinsic motivation comes from outside the individual, most often in the form of incentives. Typically a contingent arrangement is made that if you succeed, then you get these things—more pay, promotions, honors, rewards, benefits, or special privileges. The message is that if you succeed here is what you get. While this formula is sufficient to motivate many individuals, there are two serious limitations. Firstly, the person may not be that interested in the incentives to begin with, and, secondly, the incentives can only be delivered after the person has completed the task. However, if the person does not get started in the first place, the incentives are left hanging out there somewhere, comparable to a buffet banquet with no one taking a plate and helping themselves to the meal.

Intrinsic Motivation

Intrinsic motivation has its roots in *internal* factors. These factors, by contrast with external incentives, address the individual at personal or inner levels and are much more difficult to identify and put into action. Intrinsic motivators directly address:

- self-respect

- personal pride

- the experience of taking control of things in one's own way, "I did it" or "I am doing it"

- the experience of success as a function of one's own efforts

- self-satisfaction

- self-esteem

- the focus on mastery versus tangible recognition items for success.

- self-actualization, the belief in self that the job can be done, "I can do this."

The emphasis in this chapter, and throughout this book, is to take concrete steps to assist the individual with alcoholism to focus on steps for attaining *intrinsic motivation.*

Motivation for the Alcoholic

Given these two broad divisions, intrinsic and extrinsic, motivation becomes a *formidable challenge* for the alcoholic. The reason is that neither extrinsic nor intrinsic motivation can readily help an alcoholic make a commitment to undertake a lifelong recovery plan. In the first place, external motivators are not likely to motivate these individuals who have adjusted to life without these incentives. They have systematically lost interest in the normal incentives through excessive drinking. They have been willing to sacrifice jobs, income, relationships, and success through their addiction to drinking. Consequently, these incentives have already been dismissed or diminished. Additional incentives are usually ineffective after the person has become an alcoholic because the need for alcohol is so strong that other incentives cannot compete. Similarly, through the effects of alcoholism, individuals not only experience a loss of control over alcohol but a loss of control over most aspects of their lives. As a result, it is often fruitless trying to address internal factors such as self-esteem or personal pride when these core values have been systematically eroded through ongoing relinquishment of control to alcohol. Alcoholics typically do not believe they can succeed in becoming sober.

While the task of securing a commitment from the alcoholic is obviously challenging, there exist countless success stories from alcoholics who have made such a commitment. It can be done. Unfortunately, there are countless individuals who have not made such a commitment and who still suffer from the effects of alcoholism. However, we believe that many individuals can be reached through examining the details of how other alcoholics have made a commitment to making a firm decision to get onboard with a solid recovery plan.

Ten Factors Enabling Alcoholics to Make a Commitment

While it is very difficult for alcoholics to make a decision to quit drinking and undertake a recovery plan, it is not impossible. Many alcoholics have already made such a decision and are enjoying the lifelong benefits of restored sobriety. As mentioned earlier, one way for an alcoholic to make this necessary commitment, or for professionals to assist the alcoholic with this decision, is to carefully identify and review factors that have enabled other alcoholics to successfully quit drinking. By making such a review, the alcoholic may identify with the reasons given and conclude that if one alcoholic can make the leap, so can another. The success of others who have faced similar circumstances helps to give alcoholics hope—it can be done. Ten common reasons for making a commitment to quit drinking given by alcoholics are: 1. Admission of a problem, 2. "Bottoming Out," 3. Crisis wake-up call, 4. Realizing their drinking cannot be controlled, 5. Encounter with an acquaintance in recovery, 6. Allaying fear of alcohol withdrawal problems, 7. Intervention of family members or close friends, 8. Reviewing benefits of sobriety, 9. Taking graduated steps to self-control, and 10. Presence of warning signs.

Factor 1: Admission of a Problem

Alcoholism has been described as a progression beginning with social drinking which can, in approximately 1 out of 16 cases, lead to alcoholism (Jellinik, 1960). A social drinker needing to escape social problems can reach an early stage of alcoholism by the need to escape problems and is characterized by *denial* of excessive drinking. In due course tolerance for alcohol increases and the individual drinks more and more resulting in late stage alcoholism where many severe or crisis situations arise (more detail on this progression will be provided in Chapter 4, Detoxification). The whole progression of alcoholism has its roots in denial, sneaky behavior, lying, and anger and resentment when references are made to drinking issues. Consequently, the very first step toward recovery, making commitment to quit alcohol, requires the individual to *admit* that he or she has a drinking problem that is out of control. In effect, the individual must say "I am an alcoholic and I need help." If this direct admission and acceptance of the problem is absent, or demurred to any extent, successful long term recovery is not likely.

Factor 2: "Bottoming Out"

The old adage "Things will get worse before they can get better," certainly applies to alcoholism. The personal cost to alcoholics as a function of their drinking just gets worse and worse. Many experience serious health issues, lose their careers, savings, relationships, their dreams, and, above all, lose any sense of self-worth or pride. They degenerate from drinking high-end scotch to the cheapest and strongest beer or wine they can get. In a painfully real sense they "hit rock bottom." Some alcoholics have to reach this point before they are willing to do something about their problem and get help.

Factor 3: Crisis Wake-Up Call

The process of "bottoming out" is gradual. However, some alcoholics may respond to a single event that has a significant impact on their lives, such as the publicity given to a drunken driving incident or tragedy; legal proceedings against them; loss of custody of children; being served notice of divorce proceedings; being fired from employment; receiving feedback from a doctor on imminent health issues such as heart or liver problems; or the sudden death of a drinking buddy due to excessive alcohol use. These crisis events can trigger resolve for alcoholics to do something about their drinking problems—the crises serves as a "wake up call."

Factor 4: Realizing Their Drinking Cannot be Controlled

Alcoholics are masters of denial and delusion when it comes to taking the necessary steps to quit drinking. Alcohol counselors, support staff, families, and friends have heard every excuse in the book for why the alcoholic does not need to quit, or is in the process of quitting. Many alcoholics basically believe that being drunk, specifically the repercussions from being drunk, is the real problem rather than the drinking of alcohol, hence the alcoholic focuses on how to control drinking as opposed to how to quit drinking. Most alcoholics believe they can control their drinking habits and try one thing after another to establish control, such as drinking after certain hours, drinking only on weekends, restricting the number of glasses consumed, alternating alcohol with glasses of water, avoiding certain places or acquaintances, matching money spent on alcohol with some other fund, switching to light beer or low-calorie alcoholic drinks; using taller glasses for mixed drinks so more ice or soft drink can be used, and so it goes. At a certain point some alcoholics will say "I have run out of ideas to control my drinking. I am not succeeding." Or, some may go further and conclude that they cannot control their drinking—their drinking controls them. This stark realization can precipitate the need for an individual to make a commitment to quit alcohol or to get help to quit.

Factor 5: Encounter with an Acquaintance in Recovery

Alcoholics often have fixed routines, where and when they drink, which means that they often associate with other alcoholics who have similar patterns. It sometimes happens that alcoholics will run into someone with whom they used to drink who has disappeared for some time. It so happens that this person has quit drinking and has established a whole new lifestyle. The alcoholic may be struck by changes that are obviously present with the person in recovery. The person may have lost weight, assumed a better skin coloration, looks much calmer, and in control. The alcoholic may say, "You look great. What have you been up to?" The person in recovery can speak freely about quitting alcohol and of the benefits obtained. "I quit alcohol and am doing much better now. I feel better and am enjoying life." A chance encounter like this can make alcoholics think more about their own situation and be encouraged by what this acquaintance has accomplished with the implication that "If he or she can do it, so can I."

Factor 6: Allaying Fear of Alcohol Withdrawal Problems

One of the biggest threats facing an alcoholic considering quitting is fear that the withdrawal effects will be too severe to manage. Alcoholics at the late stage of alcoholism may be aware that alcohol withdrawal symptoms can lead to hospitalization or even death. An alcoholic has already experienced a substantial erosion of self-control and the idea that quitting leads to severe suffering may be enough to keep the individual drinking. Alcoholics, at earlier stages in the progression may fear what friends may think or feel shame at having to be treated as an alcoholic. Ideally, persons who are in positions to help alcoholics understand that the alcohol withdrawal symptoms cannot be minimized or sugar coated. Alcoholics must understand the need to "cowboy up" or "pony up" to a tough process in which the combination of their own resolve and the ongoing support that is available will lead to success. More detail is provided on the subject of managing alcohol withdrawal symptoms in Chapter 4, Detoxification. In general, although alcoholics may fear withdrawal symptoms, they need to be fully informed of the help they can be given to effectively cope with these effects once they make the decision to quit drinking and become sober.

Factor 7: Intervention of Family Members or Close Friends

One of the greatest sources of help for an alcoholic comes from the persistent urgings of family and close friends. Generally, when alcoholics are challenged on their excessive drinking they retort, "I'm not hurting anyone but myself!" The family can then respond that they are being hurt as well and that their family life is being destroyed. The close friend can say, "Look, I care about you. I hate seeing you destroying yourself like this." Family and close friends are in a unique position of being able to help alcoholics look beyond themselves to the wellbeing of others. This shift of focus can lead individuals to take stock of themselves and reflect on the havoc that their behavior is causing the very ones they care for and who care for them.

Factor 8: Reviewing Benefits of Sobriety

For some individuals it may be helpful to identify all the factors that would make one consider giving up drinking. The list of benefits would include issues concerning career, family and social outcomes, reduction of health related problems, becoming more productive and involved, or any other issues that one knows would get resolved if one were to give up drinking. It can be helpful to prepare a personal list of these benefits to be read and reflected on at intervals throughout the day. Copies can be posted in strategic places, like the refrigerator, the bathroom shaving mirror, or any other similar place. What this does is to keep the benefits of sobriety before the individual and may help the alcoholic to make the leap to quit drinking and get whatever help is needed.

Factor 9: Taking Graduated Steps to Self-Control

The cornerstone of alcoholism is *loss of control.* Consequently, once a person loses control over alcohol, a major result is a loss of control of in many other areas. The person can become "beaten." So when confronted with the weighty decision to quit drinking, the alcoholic does not have the resourcefulness or self-confidence to make the decision to quit nor the confidence to address all that is involved with such a decision. For some individuals it is helpful to begin to experience taking control of certain things which we might consider other steps because these steps are attainable. For example, the alcoholic could begin to make certain decisions—making a time to meet someone; developing a little plan to clean house, such as the bedroom today, the living room tomorrow; developing a schedule for the morning, the day, or the week (whichever is attainable); sitting down and making a menu for the day or week. These small, day-to-day decisions will help alcoholics gradually take charge of their day, begin to sense they are making decisions, following through, and experiencing success as a direct result of their efforts. By taking these graduated steps to get back some control, the alcoholic is in a stronger position to make the bigger step to quit alcohol and follow a path to recovery.

Factor 10: Presence of Warning Signs

Alcoholics typically become quite adept in denying they have a problem with alcohol even though others can clearly see significant issues or warning signs. One way to help alcoholics begin to address these problems is to assist them in assessing the warning signs they have. These warning signs have been well documented and are presented in Form 3.1: Checklist for Warning Signs for Alcoholism (Appendix A).

> **Note:** There is no assumption that these ten factors listed above are exhaustive. The alcoholic, or support staff person, may identify other factors that

contribute to the decision of making a commitment to quit alcohol and become sober.

Checklists and Action Plan

Two checklists and an action plan are described: 1. Checklist for warning signs of alcoholism, and 2. Checklist and action plan for committing to quit alcohol.

Checklist for Warning Signs of Alcoholism

A comprehensive checklist is presented in Appendix A: Form 3.1, Checklist for Warning Signs of Alcoholism, located at the back of the book in the appendices section. An example of a completed form is presented in Illustration 3.1.

The person can complete the checklist for warning signs, Form 3.1, independently or can make the responses in the presence of a counselor or support person. The checklist items use the personal pronouns "I," "me," and "my," which help some individuals make a more personal and honest response.

Here are some guidelines for completing the checklist:

1. It is helpful to have the individual read all the checklist items through aloud (1–13) before responding.

2. The scoring is set up as *Yes* or *No*. We have experienced many individuals preferring to respond with "Don't know" or "Maybe," which is again part the denial practice. If the response is clearly *Yes* or clearly *No*, then make the response accordingly. If the person is unsure, then the response is to be written as *Yes*.

3. It is important individuals put down their initial response to the question on the checklist. This first response is the most reliable and most honest.

4. The individual is encouraged to describe each *Yes* response in the Explanations column of the checklist. This step helps to ensure there is some reasoning behind why the person chose *Yes*.

Background: Dennis is a 46-year-old high school teacher, married with two children. He has worked at this job since college. The small town in which he lives is a farming community and his public drinking has not called attention to itself. However, his private drinking and his frequenting bars in the neighboring towns have been noticed and comments have been made. His wife, while not quite threatening divorce, is most upset with his drinking. He was in college when he began drinking, and he quickly became a regular in bars. He is a daily drinker now and he sneaks drinks.

ILLUSTRATION 3.1: Checklist for Warning Signs of Alcoholism

Factor	Applicable (Underline) **Yes No** (Maybe is a Yes)	Explanations of Yes Responses
1. Do I drink alone when I feel stressed, angry, or depressed?	<u>Yes</u> No	Describe how often: *I feel stressed, angry, or depressed, most days. I drink every day.*
2. Do I make or find excuses to drink?	<u>Yes</u> No	Name some excuses I use: *The rowdy kids at school, lack of money, nagging wife, boredom—nothing else to do in this town.*
3. Does my drinking make me late for work?	<u>Yes</u> No	Describe how often and what happened: *I am always losing my keys, billfold, or I can't find my brief case. I go back to sleep after the alarm goes off and my wife won't wake me up anymore. I am late once or twice a week.*
4. Has my family said they are worried about my drinking?	<u>Yes</u> No	Describe what they said or did: *My wife is always going on about that I drink just like her father who died in a car wreck while he was drinking. She complains we have no money and that I waste what we have on booze.*
5. Do I drink after telling myself I won't?	<u>Yes</u> No	Describe the most recent example: *Last Friday I was going to go straight home but my last class was totally stressful so I stopped just for a couple. I ended up leaving the bar at 10 pm.*
6. When I set limits on my drinking, do I fail to keep them?	<u>Yes</u> No	Describe the most recent occurrence: *Yesterday I swore I'd have just two beers but I got into a discussion about the upcoming elections and stayed and drank for 3 hours.*
7. Do I have trouble remembering things I did while drinking?	Yes <u>No</u>	Describe an instance: *I had a blackout when I was 20 or so but that is all.*
8. Do I have headaches, stomach upsets, the shakes, or hangovers the next morning after drinking?	<u>Yes</u> No	Describe ill effects of the most recent example: *The other morning I had to leave a class to throw up. I am aware my hands shake mostly on the weekends. I have really bad headaches then as well.*

ILLUSTRATION 3.1: *Continued*

9. Do I find I am drinking daily to function?	Yes	<u>No</u>	Describe: *I function just fine. I do drink every day but so does everyone else that I know.*
10. Do I get angry when confronted about drinking?	<u>Yes</u>	No	Describe the last example: *Well, I get angry about my wife going on about it. She blames any problem on my drinking.*
11. Have my eating habits changed much from drinking?	<u>Yes</u>	No	Describe in what way they have changed: *The only thing I can think about is I have to watch what I eat for the first meal of the day. It goes right through me often.*
11. Am I taking less care of my physical appearance**?**	<u>Yes</u>	No	Describe any changes: *I'm always in a rush to get to school and often miss having a shower.*
12. Have I had health changes or issues recently?	Yes	<u>No</u>	Describe these health issues: *I'm okay here.*
13. Other	<u>Yes</u>	No	Explain: *Drinking used to give me a buz and make me happy. Now I just seem to drink.*

SCORING: Total Number of *Yes* Scores: <u> 11 </u>   Total Number of *No* Scores: <u> 3 </u>

CONCLUSION

• Score of *Yes* to any item should be addressed. There may be a problem with alcohol.

• Score of 2 or more *Yes* items means <u>there most likely is a serious problem with alcohol and help should be obtained (see a doctor and address drinking)</u>.
There is definitely a problem with alcohol.

Source: Adapted from http://www.mysobriety.com/physical_effects.html; http://signsofalcoholism.org.

Checklist and Action Plan for Committing to Quit Alcohol

We know from human behavior in general that there is often quite a gap between entertaining an idea, however good it is, and translating that idea into action. A Chinese proverb aptly says: "Vision without action is a dream." The development of a checklist and action plan assists the alcoholic in translating ideas into action since recovery from alcoholism must involve *action*. Throughout Sections Two and Three, where the focus is on strategies and recovery plans, a checklist and action plan will be provided at the end of each chapter. The purpose is to assist the reader, who may be an alcoholic or a professional support person assisting an alcoholic, to evaluate the situation, list specific relevant issues, and develop an action plan.

The purpose of this checklist and action plan is to help an alcoholic reflect on issues related to making a commitment to quit alcohol and undertake a recovery plan. The ten factors described earlier in this chapter items described in Chapter 3 for assisting with decision making are listed along with a *Yes/No* response based on the relevance of the item to the alcoholic, followed by specific explanations for the items that have been responded to as *Yes*. The lower half of the form is a fill-in action plan on how the individual will use the information from the top half of the form. A blank form for the checklist, Appendix B: Form 3.2, Checklist and Action Plan for Committing to Quit Alcohol, is presented in the appendices section. An example of Form 3.2 is described in Illustration 3.2.

Background: Continuing with Dennis (Illustration 3.1) who had 11 warning signs of alcohol problem.

ILLUSTRATION 3.2: Checklist and Action Plan for Committing to Quit Alcohol

Factor	Applicable (Underline) Yes or No	Explanation
1. Have I admitted that I have a drinking problem I cannot control?	<u>Yes</u> No	*Consciously I think that this day I won't drink or I will have just one or two drinks but once I start I don't stop until I run out of money or time. Looks like I can't control my drinking.*
2. Have I "bottomed out?"	<u>Yes</u> No	*I guess. I just have run out of plans. No matter what strategy I try I fail and I drink.*
3. Have I experienced a crisis wake-up call?	<u>Yes</u> No	*Last Monday night my wife locked me out of the house and I could not fit the key in the lock. As I sat on the porch it hit me that things have gotten real serious.*
4. Have I tried everything to control my drinking and failed?	<u>Yes</u> No	*I have tried to limit my drinks or spend so much only; to drink only on weekends. I worked out at the gym. I even started going to prayer meetings at church. I'm done—nothing is working.*
5. Have I encountered an acquaintance successfully in recovery?	<u>Yes</u> No	*At the beginning of the school year I met a new teacher who was in AA. I have talked to him about drinking in general a few times. He is a good listener.*

ILLUSTRATION 3.2: Continued

6. Do I have fears about alcohol withdrawal problems?	<u>Yes</u>	No	*I marked yes but I believe it is more concern than fear. I really do not know what to expect.*
7. Have family members or close friends intervened with me?	<u>Yes</u>	No	*Not intervened so much. My parents and my wife certainly nag about my drinking. A colleague at school thought I might have a problem. Someone left an AA pamphlet on my desk at school.*
8. Have I closely reviewed the benefits of sobriety?	Yes	<u>No</u>	*To tell the truth I have not thought that far ahead.*
9. Have I taken graduated steps to self-control?	Yes	<u>No</u>	*No. Not apart from the steps I took to control drinking (which didn't work)*
10. Are there warning signs (from Form 3.1) that I have a drinking problem?	<u>Yes</u>	No	*Yes absolutely. I struck out on most of them.*
11. Are other warning signs present?	Yes	<u>No</u>	*Not that I am aware of but there probably are as I scored so high on the listed ones.*

ACTION PLAN

State with reasons what your present decision is regarding making a commitment to quit drinking and undertake a recovery plan.

I commit to doing what it takes. I talked to Bill my sober friend and he agreed that I have a drinking problem and that he would help me become sober. So I have decided that no matter what I am not going to take another drink. I have called Bill every night and take my lunch with him during the day. He has given me this book and I have been reading that at night. I have told my wife that I am going to start going to meetings with Bill. Actually I feel stronger having admitted that it is my drinking. I told my wife that I am going to start going to meetings with Bill and try to get sober. She was very pleased.

Chapter Summary

There appears to be universal agreement among researchers, writers, support professionals for alcoholics, family members, and friends of alcoholics that the first step in a successful recovery plan is a *full commitment* from the alcoholic. However, such a commitment is typically very difficult. By definition, alcoholism is an addiction wherein the individual has lost control. Alcohol has taken over this person's life to an extent that many have become quite powerless in dealing with the problem. To make the kind of commitment necessary, the alcoholic has to draw on a level of resourcefulness that has been systematically eroded through alcoholism.

However, all is not lost. Many alcoholics have been able to make the commitment to quit drinking and embark on lifelong recovery. An examination of factors that have enabled these recovering alcoholics to make this commitment provides critical information that can be of immeasurable help to other alcoholics. Essentially the rule is "What one alcoholic can do, so can another." These factors have been identified and described. Checklists and action plans are presented, with illustrations, to assist the alcoholic (with help from a support person as appropriate) to assess the situation and develop an action plan to likewise make a firm commitment to stop drinking and undertake a plan for a sober lifestyle.

SECTION TWO

Tools for Beginning Sobriety

Chapter 4: Tools for Detoxification
Chapter 5: Tools for Defusing Cravings
Chapter 6: Tools for Meeting Initial Needs

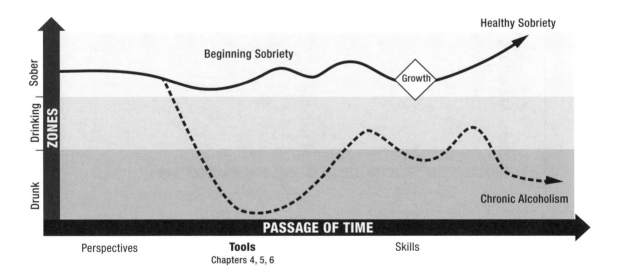

t is relatively easy to get started in becoming an alcoholic—just have a glass of alcohol, experience some benefits, and make this a routine part of one's life. For some individuals, as described in Chapter 2, these routines can then become habitual with the effects of alcohol itself becoming the driving force leading alcoholism. The purpose of this section is to carefully examine the steps needed to *release* an individual from the grip of alcoholism and to *replace* this destructive practice with lifelong constructive habits that significantly improve the person's quality of life. Simply put, this section provides tools for helping a person *become sober.*

It should be a simple matter to become sober—quit drinking. However, to free a person from alcohol use is quite a daunting challenge. When alcoholics recognize that they need to stop drinking, typically they have reached the end of their rope. That is they feel they are at rock bottom in terms of energy and are quite pessimistic about whether this all-consuming problem can be fixed or not. For them everything seems to be broken and they have no idea where to begin to salvage their lives.

In this section we present tools to help individuals navigate through the process of quitting alcohol and attaining beginning sobriety which is the first step toward recovery. The specific steps are derived from a close examination of the pathway to alcoholism as illustrated in Figure 2.5: Pathway to Alcoholism (repeated below).

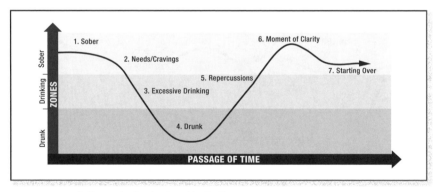

FIGURE 2.5: Pathway to Beginning Alcoholism

The first three phases, *sober, needs/cravings,* and *excessive drinking,* are the key intervention areas for targeting alcoholism. The fundamental assumption is that alcoholism has been established through a cyclical pathway. In order to break this cycle of alcoholism, the individual must establish an *alternative pathway,* that is, a *competing pathway.* Consequently, when triggers (needs and cravings) arise, instead of following the pathway of drinking alcohol leading to drunkenness, the individual engages in alternative activities that meet the person's needs in a constructive manner and thereby avert the pathway to alcoholism. In effect a *competing pathway* is established—to *beginning sobriety.*

A second perspective from Chapter 2, Figure 2.7, is that two competing pathways are available. One, the lower path, represents the pathway to chronic alcoholism (normally referred to as the alcoholic) and the other, the upper path, represents the pathway to a sober lifestyle. The idea is that individuals have a choice. They can opt for sustaining a pathway to alcoholism, or knuckle down and apply themselves

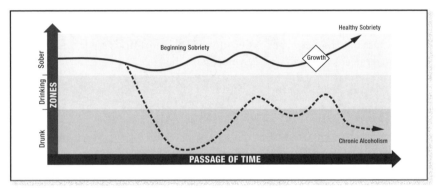

FIGURE 2.7: The Choices—Chronic Alcoholism or Healthy Sobriety

to the following steps for developing a competing pathway to a sober and healthy lifestyle.

The basic approach in this book is to describe a step-by-step process to reverse the pathway to alcoholism. To begin with, the individual must quit alcohol resulting in a new pathway called *beginning sobriety.* The tools for becoming sober have been well documented and soundly established over many years. Additional interventions will be described in Section Three for building on this beginning sobriety to attain ongoing growth toward healthy sobriety. The tools for attaining beginning sobriety target three major areas which constitute the chapters for this section: 1. Detoxification, 2. Defusing cravings, and 3. Meeting initial needs.

These tools are described in this section with procedural details, illustrations, and checklists and action plans:

Chapter 4: Tools for Detoxification. Initially, individuals already have alcohol in their system and have an established routine of drinking. So the first step involves *freeing* themselves from this routine of drinking and cleansing their system by total abstinence from alcohol.

Chapter 5: Tools for Defusing Cravings. Once the person ceases to drink alcohol, cravings set in causing considerable discomfort. These cravings must be managed effectively.

Chapter 6: Tools for Meeting Initial Needs. The initial needs, triggers, were temporarily met through the consumption of alcohol will re-emerge once the person becomes sober. Now, individuals must find *replacement* activities to meet needs that arise as they become sober.

Tools for Detoxification

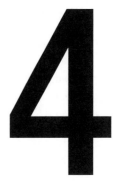

Going to Hell is easy; it's coming back that's hard.

— *The Aeneid*, Virgil

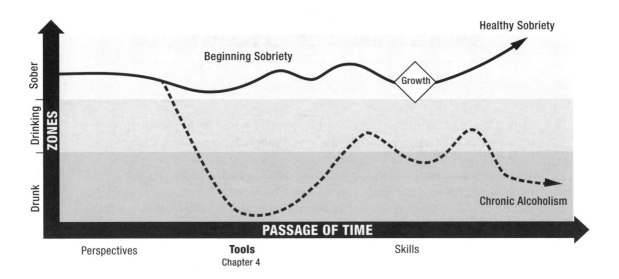

O nce a person has made a firm commitment to address his or her alcoholism, the next question is where to start. Individuals who examine published literature and online information on how to treat alcoholism will more than likely be overwhelmed with the wide array of strategies, suggestions, treatment plans, and institutional assistance programs. While each of these approaches may differ substantially in their basic philosophy, they share one thing in common when it comes to addressing alcoholism—alcohol consumption must cease entirely.

A common pathway to alcoholism has been presented in terms of seven phases: 1. Sober, 2. Needs/Cravings, 3. Excessive drnking , 4. Drunk, 5. Repercussions, 6. Moment of clarity, and 7. Starting over (see Figure 2.5, repeated from Chapter 2).

> **The individual must quit alcohol—Totally, immediately, and unconditionally.**

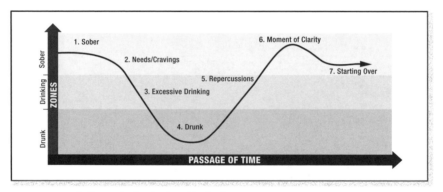

FIGURE 2.5: Pathway to Beginning Alcoholism

Typically, excessive drinking becomes the normal response to the prevailing unmet needs and cravings which lead to drunkenness, repercussions, and the cycle continues. This book, along with the majority of programs for addressing alcoholism, takes the position that before any lifelong changes can occur for alcoholics, *the pathway to alcoholism must be terminated.* After this, an alternative pathway, a sharp detour if you will, to a constructive and healthy lifestyle can then be established.

The first intervention in this process is depicted in Figure 4.1: Tools for Detoxification. A large X is inserted in the Sober zone on the graph well before Phase 3, Excessive Drinking. The idea is that the pathway to alcoholism stops right here—no more drinking. The broken line in Figure 4.1 indicates the beginning of the detoxification process; X represents the dissolution of this pathway—no more drinking, no more drunkenness, no more repercussions, and no more starting over.

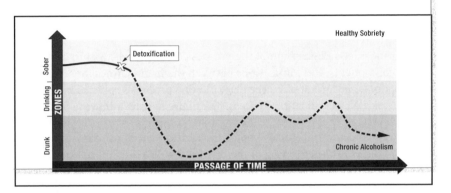

FIGURE 4.1: Tools for Detoxification

The stage is being set for a detour to a new pathway that leads to a healthy, stable, and sober lifestyle. The Drinking and Drunk zones are circumvented.

This first step of quitting alcohol may sound quite straight forward. *Emphatically, this is not the case,* especially for hard core alcoholics. When a full-fledged alcoholic ceases to drink alcohol, effects known as *alcohol withdrawal symptoms* come into play immediately. These effects can have a range of problems depending on the severity or level of alcoholism. For the low level alcoholics the effects are short-term discomfort. For the high level, fully fledged alcoholic the effects can be quite distressing, traumatic, and occasionally catastrophic for the individual if sufficient care is not taken.

This process where an individual ceases to consume alcohol and the immediate effects of alcohol withdrawal symptoms are addressed is called *detoxification,* the subject of this chapter. The term detoxification is derived from the word *toxin* because of the negative effects alcohol has on the body, especially for the major organs, heart, liver, and kidneys. Consequently, these toxins need to be removed as a critical first step in a lifelong recovery plan from alcoholism.

The detoxification process involves the interaction of three important components which must be properly understood and thoroughly planned for in advance. These interacting components include:

1. The progression of alcoholism

2. The levels of alcohol withdrawal symptoms

3. The continuum of treatment options

This chapter includes a description of the progressions, or levels, within each of these three components, the connections between them, guidelines for selecting treatment options, and an exit plan. The detoxification process is depicted in Figure 4.2: Components of the Detoxification Process. The figure has the following features:

- The first and a most critical event is the medical check-up shown in the box in boldface at the beginning of the continuum of treatment options.

- The three components are presented as three separate columns with different shapes for each component.

- The block arrows pointing downward connect the stages or levels *within* each of the three components.

- The shape for each of these stages and levels decreases in size representing the decreasing numbers of persons trying to quit at a particular stage and the decreasing numbers of persons experiencing symptoms at a particular level. For example, most alcoholics, 80–90%, represented by the largest hexagon, are at Stage I, *Early,* while the fewest, 3–5%, are at Stage III, Late, represented by the smallest hexagon. Although, the more serious symptoms occur at Level III and the least serious at Level I, Level I applies to more people than Level III hence the largest square is used for Level I.

- The solid line arrows connecting the components depict the most common pathway *between* the components. For example, those alcoholics in the Early stage of alcoholism are likely to experience the alcoholic withdrawal symptoms of Level I, Tremors, while the Late stage alcoholics are likely to experience the third level, Delirium Tremens (DTs).

- The broken line arrows connecting the components depict a *possible* pathway *between* the components. For example, an individual alcoholic at an Early stage of alcoholism may experience the withdrawal symptoms of Level II, Hallucinations, Tremors, and Petit Seizures. The most common pathway is shown by the solid line arrows but treatment supervisors and support personnel must always be ready for the less common pathway.

• The final component, Exit Plan, is depicted as a diamond and is linked to each of the three treatment plans. The strong recommendation is that regardless of the type of treatment plan the individual selects, there should be a clear exit or discharge plan.

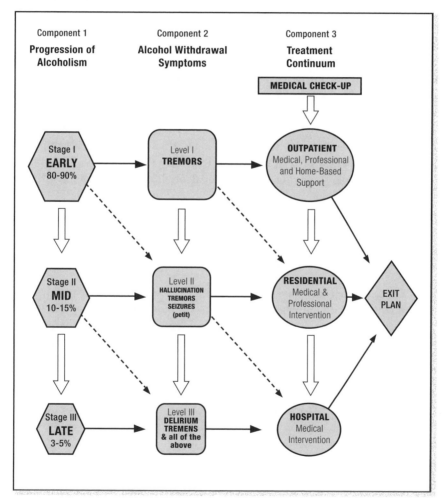

FIGURE 4.2: Components of the Detoxification Process

Component 1: The Progression of Alcoholism

(Represented by hexagons in the first column of Figure 4.2)

More than likely the first question alcoholics will ask when they decide to quit alcohol is "What's going to happen to me?" Typically alcoholics are somewhat aware of the problems associated with alcohol withdrawal and may have heard some horror stories from others who have quit drinking. Clearly, it is very important for alcoholics to understand that the effects of alcohol withdrawal are related to the specific stages of alcoholism. The preparation and level of treatment an individual alcoholic may need are determined by the particular stage of alcoholism the individual has reached.

The pioneer work on stages of alcoholism or alcoholic progression has been widely attributed to Jellinek (1960). A key concept in his work became known as the Jellinek Curve. Jellinek introduced the idea of classification of alcoholics based on the stages or progression levels of alcoholism from its earliest stages through various levels to the most advanced or late stage. Of particular importance in this model is that alcoholics are not regarded as one group of people requiring one treatment. Rather the model classifies alcoholics according to the severity of their symptoms which in turn defines the level of support or treatment the person needs. For the purposes of this book, three stages or levels of alcoholic progression will be used: early stage, mid-stage, and late stage.

Early Stage

(Represented by the largest hexagon in Figure 4.2)

In the *early stage* the individual has progressed from social drinking to drinking more frequently and imbibing greater quantities compared to their associates in the social drinking network. Their tolerance for alcohol substantially increases and the need to consume greater amounts of alcohol increases. The drinking is typically driven by confidence issues and needs, for relief from stress, or to escape from problems, and in some cases the need for ongoing enhancement—the need to feel better and have more fun. Associated with increased drinking, the individual experiences regular hangovers, forgetfulness, resents references to his or her drinking excesses, becomes sneakier about drinking routines, and in some cases may pass out.

Mid-Stage
(Represented by the medium-sized hexagon in Figure 4.2)

At *mid-stage* cravings for alcohol set in and the individuals *must drink* regardless of the time or cost. The individuals experience significant loss of control over alcohol consumption in terms of time, place, and amount of drinking. People at this stage often drink in the morning to help take care of hangovers from drinking the evening before. Often at this stage the individuals make various attempts to control their drinking such as changing locations or drinking with different people. These changes made at mid-stage, however, tend to be unsuccessful in controlling the drinking.

Late Stage
(Represented by the smallest hexagon in Figure 4.2)

By the *late stage* the person has lost all control over alcohol and has become a loner in drinking with significant changes occurring in personal relationships, work

> **There are two very clearly related trends in reviewing this three-stage progression in alcoholism:**
>
> - A rapid loss of control over drinking from marginal control initially to no control in the late stage.
>
> - A clear deterioration in health and general functioning for the individual from beginning problems to life-threatening concerns.

sites, and community relationships. Many serious physical changes occur such as the shakes, delirium, hallucinations, malnutrition, and internal stress on organs (especially the heart, liver, and kidneys). The individual is now very high risk for serious health issues. The person drinks solely for the sake of drinking. Frequent binges occur which ultimately may lead to serious health problems which could lead to death in some cases.

Component 2: Alcohol Withdrawal Symptoms
(Represented by squares in the second column of Figure 4.2)

The effects of quitting alcohol on an individual are called *alcohol withdrawal symptoms* (represented by squares in the middle column of Figure 4.2). When a person decides to quit drinking, or is in the process of making such a decision, it is absolutely essential that these accompanying symptoms are properly understood in order for a safe and successful recovery plan to be developed, implemented and sustained. The following topics are addressed in this section: a. The nature of alcohol withdrawal symptoms, b. The levels of alcohol withdrawal symptoms, and c. Determining what to expect.

Nature of Alcohol Withdrawal Symptoms

The alcoholic, friend, or family member may well ask, "Why should we expect immediate problems, or withdrawal problems, when an alcoholic quits alcohol?" The answer lies in the nature of *dependency*. Once a person becomes an alcoholic, the individual begins to crave alcohol and the body demands alcohol like a tyrant. The person has to sustain drinking in order to meet these physical and emotional needs of the body. The person must have alcohol to obtain calm and stability (albeit short term). Literally, there is no relief until alcohol starts flowing through the system. Alcohol has become a critical need for the individual.

Now when the individual quits alcohol, the body it is not getting what it needs, so it begins to strongly react. If the person shakes prior to drinking, then he or she will shake much more when the drinking is denied. If the individual becomes agitated prior to drinking, then the agitation will substantially escalate when drinking does not occur. The body essentially "rebels" when denied alcohol, and this rebellion can take many forms including significant changes in emotions involving anger, depression, and frustration; mental instability with serious lapses in judgment, communication, and focus; and, moreover, for advanced cases of alcoholism, serious health problems can arise such as becoming unconscious and life-threatening heart and vital organ damage can occur.

These alcohol withdrawal symptoms are quite analogous to an *extinction burst* described in behavioral literature. Basically, individuals are often rewarded by using certain behaviors to gain something or to establish control, such as by yelling, bullying, or using violence. However, if the rewards are removed *(extinction)*, the individual will escalate to regain the reward by yelling more, bullying more, or using more violence *(extinction burst)*. In the same way, when the cycle of alcoholism is interrupted through not drinking, the whole person becomes more agitated and reacts more strongly. The person is used to having alcohol and when cut off *(extinction)* significant reactions are likely to occur *(extinction burst)*.

There is also a progression regarding the extent or seriousness of the alcohol withdrawal symptoms which are directly linked to the specific stage of the individual's progression with alcoholism. An individual at an early stage of alcoholism might expect less severe withdrawal symptoms compared to one at the late stage. This progression of alcohol withdrawal symptoms is characterized by levels.

Levels of Alcohol Withdrawal Symptoms
(Represented by squares of different sizes in Figure 4.2)

It is clear that not all alcoholics experience the same levels of alcohol withdrawal symptoms when they quit alcohol. As mentioned, the effects the individuals experience will be determined by the respective stage of alcoholism reached. For example, a person in the early stage of alcoholism normally experiences fewer withdrawal problems such as tremors, loss of appetite, and headaches, while a person in the late stage of alcoholism may experience profound confusion, breathing problems, and perhaps cardiovascular disturbances. The individual in the former case could be treated as an outpatient or in a limited residential care facility whereas the latter individual typically needs hospitalization.

This range of problems in the alcohol withdrawal symptoms column depicted in Figure 4.2: Components of the Detoxification Process can be categorized in terms of *three levels:* Level I, Tremors; Level II, Hallucinations, Tremors, and Petit Seizures; and Level III, All of the above plus Delirium Tremens (DTs). These levels are not designed as a progression in the sense that an individual can move from one level to the next as in the case of the stages of alcoholism. Rather the stages are presented more as *levels* or categories representing the most likely withdrawal symptoms an individual is likely to experience based on the individual's medical history and the stage reached with alcoholism.

Determining What to Expect

Level I, Tremors (represented by the largest square in Figure 4.2) is typically experienced by approximately 90% of alcoholics attempting to quit drinking and peaks around 24–36 hours after the last drink. It is characterized by:

- shakes or jitters
- irritability, uneasiness

- nausea, vomiting

- excessive urinating, flushes

- increased heart rate, blood pressure, and temperature

- loss of appetite, slurred speech, headaches, insomnia

- inattentiveness, poor coordination

Level II, Hallucinations, Tremors, and Seizures (represented by the medium-sized square in Figure 4.2) is typically experienced by approximately 15–25% of alcoholics. The withdrawal symptoms often encountered are:

- visual and auditory hallucinations

- presence of odors and sounds

- fear

- disorientation, irritability

- denial or failure to admit presence of hallucinations

- reappearance of cravings

- desire to leave or escape (presumably to renew drinking)

- seizure activity (petit mal)

- tremors and other symptoms associated with the earlier stage

Level III, All of the Above Plus Delirium Tremens, DTs, (represented by the smallest square in Figure 4.2) usually occurs 3–5 days after the last drink and can last up to 72 hours. This level is characterized by:

- symptoms associated with Levels I and II

- profound confusion

- deep hallucinations and delusions

- severe agitation, sleeplessness

- perspiration and fever

- cardiovascular disturbances which could be fatal

- increases in blood pressure, dehydration

- difficulties in breathing, circulation, and temperature control

- grand mal seizures, strokes

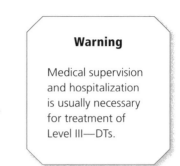

Warning

Medical supervision and hospitalization is usually necessary for treatment of Level III—DTs.

Component 3: Treatment Continuum
(Represented by the ovals in the third column of Figure 4.2)

As expected, the treatment options for managing the alcohol withdrawal symptoms match the individual's stage of alcoholism and anticipated corresponding level of alcohol withdrawal symptoms. One immediate problem in determining which stage of treatment an alcoholic may need is to have accurate information on the individual's current level of health and which alcoholic withdrawal symptoms are likely to be experienced. *First and foremost the alcoholic should go to the doctor for a physical check-up* to help determine the most appropriate treatment option.

There are basically three treatment options in the detoxification process based on the level of support needed to address the anticipated alcohol withdrawal symptoms and to effectively plan for ongoing recovery: a. Home based and outpatient, b. Residential, and c. Hospital.

Home-Based or Outpatient Treatment
(Represented by the largest oval in Figure 4.2)

In home-based treatment, individuals decide to "bite the bullet," quit drinking, and take care of the matter at home alone or with support from family or friends. Many alcoholics prefer to go this route because of their financial situation, pride factors where they believe they can take care of the problem and do not want to admit to themselves or others they are undergoing detoxification, or they are together enough to manage the responsibilities themselves. The person may be informed of the possible withdrawal effects and develop some readiness for dealing with these symptoms. It is strongly recommended that even if individuals decide to go it alone that they have *a medical checkup with their doctor before beginning the detoxification process* and that they inform or involve a family member or friend. In this way, some level of monitoring is in place to help if problems arise.

Outpatient is the typical medical or consulting model in which the patient goes to the doctor or therapist for treatment by appointment and then goes home. In this model the alcoholic takes care of most of the monitoring and adaptations needed by regularly checking in with a professional counselor or medical doctor during the process and as part of the exit plan.

Residential Treatment
(Represented by the medium-sized oval in Figure 4.2)

Residential treatment involves living in a facility for 24 hours or more so that the appropriate level of supervision and support can be provided. These facilities typically have professional staff on board who can provide consultation and support for emotional and mental withdrawal symptoms and can assist with developing an exit plan to help the individual remain sober. In addition the staff is usually well informed and able to recognize signs where medical intervention may be needed. Medical and emergency help is usually readily accessible at residential programs.

Hospital Treatment
(Represented by the smallest oval in Figure 4.2)

Hospital options are required for alcoholics beginning the detoxification step who have significant health issues to begin with, such as heart, liver, seizure activity, or kidney problems. Also, if the alcoholic is in the late stage of alcoholism, severe alcoholic withdrawal problems are expected which have a high likelihood of causing trauma and life-threatening effects. In some cases specific drugs are administered in the detoxification process. Clearly, these interventions must have medical direction and supervision.

In general, medical supervision and immediate access to treatment, available in hospital placements, is necessary for the alcoholics who are at risk with physical pre-conditions or who are in the late stages of alcoholism. In addition, hospital programs typically have a clear exit plan for the individual to follow when the hospital program is completed.

Selection of Specific Detoxification Treatment Plan

Once the first two major components of the detoxification process (stages and levels of alcohol withdrawal symptoms) are properly determined, the next step in the detoxification process is to select a specific *treatment* plan for the individual alcoholic. This treatment plan is determined by the results of the physical check-up from seeing a doctor, the stage of alcoholism reached, and what level of alcohol withdrawal symptoms might be expected. Figure 4.2 shows the connection between the three components and which treatment options (in ovals) might follow.

The above information is presented as the ideal situation for an individual alcoholic. However, other factors come into play, especially finances, especially health insurance, which may determine which option is actually available for the individual. In many cases hospitalization or some residential placements may not be an option because the individual may not have the necessary finances or adequate health insurance. However, readers are strongly encouraged to closely research what options are accessible in their area and state. Some residential programs and outpatient services offer sliding fee structures. Some states have allocated funding to support programs which include the funding of free slots. In general if the ideal treatment option is not accessible, then alternative options need to be investigated through personal research and through help from local agencies and support organizations.

Developing a Short Term Exit or Discharge Plan
(Represented by the triangle in Figure 4.2)

When a person completes the detoxification plan, specifically to quit alcohol and manage the alcohol withdrawal symptoms, the next step is to address the transition from this detoxification plan to resumption of daily living without alcohol. The details of these exit or discharge plans will vary according to the level of treatment needed for the detoxification process. A late-term alcoholic, who has experienced Level III alcohol withdrawal symptoms in a hospital, will need a detailed discharge plan to assist the individual in making the transition safely and successfully. The alcoholic at an early stage of progression, who has experienced Level I alcohol withdrawal symptoms, may need a self-directed plan, or a plan with support from professionals, to remain free from alcohol and to develop productive alternatives for a sober lifestyle.

In general, the minimum or common factors in an exit plan following the detoxification process include:

- A hot-line or contact person if immediate help is needed

- Plans to avoid certain places or people where drinking alcohol is inevitable

- Empty the home of alcohol

- Identify a support group and make immediate contact

- Develop alternative routines to avoid drinking

- Have a response ready for when cravings to drink emerge

- Have a plan to address basic needs—social, diet, exercise, and activities

- Other

Note: The emphasis in an exit or discharge plan is to provide assistance and support to the individual *immediately* following the detoxification process. Just because the person has been successful in quitting alcohol on a short term basis does not mean the individual can automatically lead a life alcohol free. Long term, ongoing planning is absolutely necessary for the individual to develop a healthy, normal, and productive lifestyle free of alcohol. Skills for this for this kind of planning are presented in Chapter 5 and 6.

Chapter Summary

Published literature is replete with information on how to address alcoholism and develop lifelong plans for sobriety. While there is great variety in these approaches, there is one thing they all share: *the alcoholic must cease drinking alcohol.* However, when an alcoholic quits drinking , there are immediate adverse effects called alcohol withdrawal symptoms which can range from low level-tremors, agitation, and discomfort to traumatic life-threatening conditions. Given these serious effects, careful planning needs to take place before the alcoholic quits drinking. The process of helping a person to quit alcohol and planning for alcohol withdrawal symptoms in a safe and successful manner is called *detoxification.*

The kinds of withdrawal problems an individual may face depends on the individual's current level of health and stage of alcoholism reached. Alcoholism is progressive and there are three major stages: early, mid, and late. The stages are basically determined by the degree of control an individual has over the drinking and the impact of the drinking on his or her life. Alcohol withdrawal symptoms can also be divided into three levels characterized by increasing intensity: tremors; hallucinations, tremors, and seizures; and all of the above plus delirium tremens. The appropriate level of treatment options is determined by the results from a physical check-up and the connections between the stage of alcoholism reached and the corresponding levels of alcohol withdrawal symptoms that are likely to be experienced. When the person completes the detoxification process, an exit plan should be developed which is designed to tie down the initial transition steps from the detoxification program to maintaining sobriety.

It is expected, and strongly recommended, that following this initial exit plan a comprehensive, ongoing, and lifelong recovery plan is developed for the individual, the details of which are described in subsequent chapters of this book.

Tools for Defusing Cravings

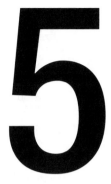

They took a drink a day or so prior to the date, and then the phenomenon of craving at once became paramount to all other interests so that the important appointment was not met. These men were not drinking to escape; they were drinking to overcome a craving beyond their mental control.

— William D. Silkworth

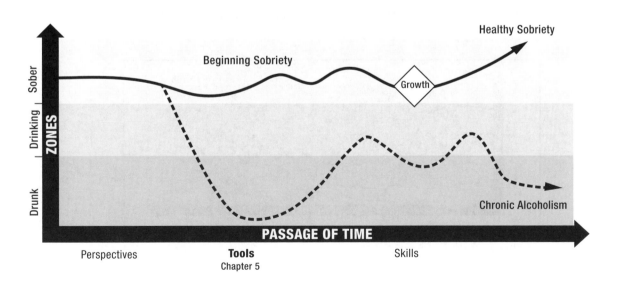

At this juncture the alcoholic has made two significant and quite valiant steps toward breaking the grip of alcoholism and establishing a pathway to sobriety. First, a firm commitment has been made to do what it takes and, second, the detoxification process of quitting alcohol and managing the alcohol withdrawal symptoms has been completed. However, the alcoholic is not out of the woods by any stretch of the imagination. The next interventions that must be addressed are to manage the *cravings* and *emerging problems* which set the stage for a new pathway to a sober lifestyle.

This chapter provides the alcoholic with tools on how to *defuse* these cravings. Chapter 2, in the development of a model to describe the pathway to alcoholism, notes that there is a progression from unmet needs, initial reasons for drinking, to cravings for alcohol. These unmet needs are those needs, experiences, circumstances, and emotional feelings that typically set the occasion for drinking alcohol. Alcohol serves to meet these needs in a relatively quick manner. Once the person begins to experience these beneficial effects of alcohol, the overall effect for some is to drink more alcohol and drink more frequently. It is only a matter of time before the effects of alcohol become the reason for drinking. The person now *must* have alcohol to calm down or relax. At this stage the person becomes an alcoholic. The unmet needs prompting drinking in the first place have now been replaced by *cravings*. Once alcohol is in the system to a significant level, cravings take over from unmet needs.

In Figure 5.1, Cravings is denoted by the large X on the graph, is essentially a continuation of intervention for detoxification.

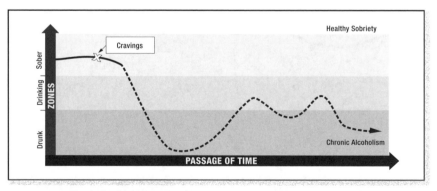

FIGURE 5.1: Tools for Defusing Cravings

The toxic effects of alcohol are still operative and are manifested as cravings which need to be defused. The broken line signifies the pathway to chronic alcoholism has been halted through the detoxification process, and defusing cravings. The alcoholic may, and will, experience, the unmet needs and cravings that typically have led the person to drinking excessively, but will now use time tested tools to manage these in such a way that drinking does not occur and that the person can now engage in activities leading to a sober lifestyle.

The approach in this book is to retrace the phases wherein alcoholism is established, backward chaining, as noted in the lead in to Section Two. The detoxification process, Chapter 4, was designated as the first set of tools for breaking up the cycle of alcoholism. Clearly excessive drinking is blocked when the person ceases to drink alcohol. The next intervention involves defusing cravings, followed by procedures for managing the emerging problems (Chapter 6). The following tools will be addressed in the development of procedures for defusing the cravings: 1. Need for planning, 2. Description of cravings, 3. Strategies to defuse cravings, and 4. Checklist and action plans.

Need for Planning

Planning for management of cravings should occur before the detoxification process begins and be maintained during and following detoxification, and well into the pathway to sobriety. As soon as an alcoholic begins the detoxification intervention, cravings will begin to operate. In fact, the individual is probably already experiencing cravings before the detoxification intervention begins.

Individuals undergoing residential treatment for detoxification, typically receive clear information on how the cravings work, what help can be given, and how they can help themselves. Usually, they are assured that help is available any time they need it, and they are encouraged to solicit help if need be.

Similarly, individuals who conduct the detoxification process themselves, or through outpatient support, should be fully informed of what to expect with cravings and on procedures for managing the cravings. The following information is a summary of what cravings are and of strategies for managing them.

Description of Cravings

Definition of Cravings

Cravings are those urges that drive a person toward drinking once they have established drinking routines. The person just has to have a drink, "I will go crazy unless I have a drink." Cravings are best characterized as *physiological needs* or *urgings*. A useful analogy is to consider cravings as a demanding appetite akin to hunger pangs. When a person really needs food, the body reacts with hunger pangs which can be manifested as stomach rumblings, cramps, shakes, headaches, restlessness, perspiration, and heart tremors in more serious cases. The message is loud and clear—the body has to eat. Similarly, with cravings for alcohol the individual may experience an array of physical symptoms all of which point to the need for alcohol. Once alcohol is consumed, these symptoms are assuaged and the individual relaxes (albeit until the alcohol has been assimilated).

Sometimes it is helpful to consider cravings as similar to the symptoms and needs displayed by persons who are afflicted with obsessive-compulsive disorders (OCD). This mental health illness is characterized by anxiety attacks that lead to irrational, ritualized, and repetitive behaviors that must be performed. These individuals are totally driven and cannot relax until their routines are completed. The cravings of an alcoholic have similar notes of urgency, anxiety, and compulsion to access alcohol.

Cue-Induced Cravings

Another dimension of cravings, which has important implications for treatment, is the notion of *cue-induced cravings* (another form of triggers to drink). Alcoholics have very set routines in limited and predictable lifestyles. They always drink at certain places, drink much the same alcohol (at least to begin with, then it is whatever they can get their hands on), drink with the same people, have the same routines, such as playing a guitar at first or pool before they settle into drinking. Because these patterns have been repeated many times, the specific routine or setting just by this association can induce cravings. For example, the person just has to see his regular tavern and the cravings for a drink take hold, or sees some pool on TV which makes him want to drink, he looks at his guitar and then feels the craving for a drink, or she sees a friend she drinks with on a regular basis and she now has to have a drink. These associations, or so called cue-induced cravings, need to be identified and addressed in the overall plan to control cravings.

Measurement of Cravings

Given individuals will be taking steps to defuse their cravings for alcohol, it is important that they have some way of determining their progress. How will they know if they are being successful or not? How will they know if their cravings have been weakened or if their cravings are coming under control? There are typically three factors involved with measuring cravings:

1. **Frequency** which simply indicates how often the cravings occur. This measure can readily be determined by keeping a log through the day and evening and noting when the cravings occur.

2. **Duration** which determines how long the cravings last. This measure can also be assessed by keeping a log and noting how long individual craving episodes last.

3. **Intensity** which measures the severity of the cravings attack. Intensity is best measured by using a scale (called a Likert-Scale) in which, for example, the individual rates the strength of the craving on a scale of 1 to 10 where a score of 1 represents a very weak craving that is barely noticeable through to a score of 10 where the craving is overpowering and severe.

Typically, the measures for cravings are highest initially, during the detoxification step, and diminish over time if concrete steps are taken to defuse them and the person totally abstains from drinking. Moreover, it is not so important to have the cravings disappear totally; rather it is important for the individual to have the tools, support from others, and confidence of mindset, to manage the cravings whenever they rear their ugly heads.

Tools for Defusing Cravings

Two areas of strategies or interventions are presented in this section: 1. Having a helpful sponsor or support person, 2. Having the right mindset, and 3. Using specific procedures for defusing cravings.

Having a Helpful Sponsor or Support Person

It is common practice among organizations that support recovering alcoholics that it is highly desirable, if not necessary in most cases, for alcoholics to be supported by a sponsor, mentor, family member, friend, and in some instances professional assistance. The reason is that alcoholics are very vulnerable at this point making it very difficult to work through the cravings alone. Cravings are powerful triggers and typically recovering alcoholics need the additional support provided by another person otherwise relapse is likely to occur.

Having the Right Mindset

The approach here refers to the understanding people have of what cravings are and how they work. By understanding the following six aspects of cravings and having an appropriate mindset or attitude toward them, the individual is in a stronger position to endure these cravings.

1. **Knowing What to Expect.** Before individuals begin the detoxification process, Chapter 4, they should be fully aware of the powerful role cravings will inevitably play. Moreover, even though the person might say "Yeah, I've been there before," it is important to understand that the cravings during detoxification, and later on, may be stronger and more drawn out because alcohol is not forthcoming. In the past when the individual had cravings, a drink always followed. The big difference now is that drinking is not an option. So the cravings will become more intense and will last longer. The idea is that "to be forewarned is to be forearmed." So, the alcoholic approaches detoxification knowing what to expect which helps to work through the cravings and quitting alcohol thereafter.

2. **It Will Get Worse Before It Gets Better.** Most of us have had surgery for something or other or at least some form of a medical procedure. The message

we are given is that there will be some pain and discomfort initially and in the case of major surgery—considerable pain. However, in time, the pain will ease and the patient will recover and be healthier as a result of the treatment. Similarly, the alcoholic needs to understand that up front there will be discomfort and, in some cases, severe cravings, but as time goes on these cravings will diminish through being alcohol free. In time the individual will come experience the benefits of being sober, which in turn will substantially weaken the cravings.

3. **Expect Uncertainty between Cravings.** The cravings are not totally continuous ("Thank goodness!" says the recovering alcoholic). This means that there will be periods of time when the person does not have cravings or there are periods between cravings. Individuals are very likely to experience uncertainty during these periods simply because it is "new territory" (unless they have had relapses and are starting again). This interlude functions like a *void*. Individuals may not know what to do here. They may feel uncertain, giddy, happy, confused, or somewhat lost and tentative. Again it is helpful to understand that this period will occur and will pass. The specific procedures for defusing cravings (presented in the following pages) are also recommended for managing these periods between cravings.

4. **It Too Shall Pass.** When individuals are experiencing cravings, especially the more intense ones, there may be feelings that "I am not going to make it." At this juncture they have to keep reminding themselves that *cravings are temporary,* they will go away. This is easy to say from a distance or outside the context, but the reality is there—the cravings will pass. Moreover, it is important to understand that cravings of themselves cannot harm you. Cravings are solely powerful *impulses* which must be ignored and which will pass away in time. The message is "Hang in there, it will pass." Again, support persons play a key role in helping the recovering alcoholic endure this period.

5. **View Cravings as Enticements or Temptations.** Some people see cravings as a "little monster" inside their mind that is trying to tempt them. It is like a voice in their mind saying, "You really need a drink," "You are not going to make it," "Look, one drink won't hurt you," "You've been real good, no beer for a week. You deserve a drink," "You have proved you can quit, so have a drink. You can quit again," and so it goes with these temptations. Some individuals find it helpful to talk back to these voices, "Get lost," "You are

not going to win this time you …" Again the individual must maintain firm resolve and stoutly resist these enticements or temptations. The support person can also help the recovering alcoholic understand and resist these temptations to drink.

6. **Realize Cravings Are a Part of Irrational Behavior.** Many people, including alcoholics, are puzzled why people would constantly drink to excess, put themselves in harm's way, and, in spite of many serious repercussions, persist with keeping drinking to excess. It does not make sense one might say. Cravings are part of this irrational behavior. Sustained harmful, irrational behavior usually leads to profound confusion and is typically resistant to rational approaches. In general, when people are faced with irrational behavior, the best approach or attitude is *just press* on, *simply do what has to be done.* For some it may be helpful to have the understanding that *I need to do this now and will sort it out later.* It is usually not helpful to try to follow the *mind's directions* as the mind will inevitably be all over the place. Do not get sidetracked. Simply focus on what has to be done and do it. It is also recommended to talk these issues through with a support person.

Using Specific Tools for Defusing Cravings

These are the concrete steps or actions a person may take when cravings arise or when cravings are anticipated. The key feature of these strategies is to help the individual *re-focus.* Cravings consume the person's attention so these strategies are designed to help shift attention away from cravings to something else and thereby weaken the hold of the cravings.

Note: There is no guarantee that any particular strategy will work for an individual who is beset with cravings. These strategies have been compiled from the literature on alcoholism, from suggestions of sponsors, and from discussions with individual alcoholics. It is up to the persons themselves to examine the strategies and select ones that might work for them. Then it is a matter of trying them out to see what helps them. Obviously, if a particular strategy is working, then keep using it. If a strategy is not helping, then try a different one. The point is to keep trying and not let the cravings prevail. The individual operates on the assumption that there is a way through this and has the resolve to find this way.

There are seven tools for assisting the recovering alcoholic to defuse cravings:

1. **Contact a Support Person.** When cravings occur, it is most important to contact a support person such as a friend, sponsor, clergy member, or relative, usually by phone, or a visit, and talk (by phone, text or instant messaging). Ideally, this contact should be set up beforehand (part of the exit plan for the initial Detoxification step) so that when the call is made the contact knows exactly why the call is being made and can respond accordingly. The subject of the conversation does not matter that much as long as they chat. Simply talking to someone else serves to provide a major distraction. Once the person being contacted understands that cravings are operating then this person can take charge of the conversation and steer it to other topics to help the alcoholic re-focus. It is best to set this up beforehand so that the contact person knows why the call is being made and that the alcoholic feels free to make the call. Contact persons need to be supportive and do their best to provide encouragement and assurances that the cravings will pass.

2. **Get Busy.** Another way of providing distractions is simply to get physically busy such as going for a walk, cleaning up the house, doing some errands, weeding the garden, going jogging, watching an engaging movie, and washing the car. Playing games with a friend such as chess, backgammon, cards, and Scrabble provide a very useful way of shifting the mind to something else. There is also an abundance of electronic games that can be accessed for individual use or to be played with a friend (it is recommended to avoid games that can lead to other addictions such as gambling games). Games also provide a conversation piece for the individual. It is helpful to have a list of such suitable activities already in mind and available, so that when the cravings emerge, the alcoholic can quickly become engaged without having to spend time mulling over what to do.

3. **Use Relaxation Techniques.** Some people prefer relaxing to getting themselves busy. Relaxation techniques are typically intended to reduce stress which, of course, includes cravings. These techniques are designed to calm down the mind and body and can have many forms, such as sitting still listening to music, sitting in silence, concentrating on one's own stillness through various forms of meditation, sitting in a quiet park and mentally shutting out the world, standing and staring at a waterfall and taking in

all the sounds, yoga, and prayer and its various forms. Controlled deep breathing is a powerful technique that often provides instant relief and can be implemented anywhere. Deep breathing helps remove tension, enables the individual to focus on the breathing versus cravings, and can be used as often as needed. There are many variations of relaxation options and the individual should carefully select ones that are more likely to suit them and work for them.

4. **Use of Symbols**. Some alcoholics always carry a symbol with them such as a coin, token, chip, flashcard, photo, or quotation. Individuals who are affiliated with religions often use a religious symbol such as rosary beads, a medal, prayer card, or religious icon. They then handle this symbol or read it when cravings arise. Similarly, the symbol can be used to help the person recite a meaningful quotation or prayer. The cravings function as temptations and the particular symbol serves as a strong reminder for what they should do or as a *don't go there* reminder.

5. **Think It Through**. For recovering alcoholics it is helpful to "talk it through" with yourself. They think or talk out loud about the consequences of drinking again, recall some of the disastrous results of past drinking episodes, such as accidents, violent sickness, hangovers, arrests, or the gradual erosion of their careers, family relationships, and personal self-worth. They ask themselves, "Is it worth it?" "Do I really want to go there again?" They then focus on their own resolve, thinking through the idea that "I have come this far and I will go further. I have made to commitment to do what it takes and by golly I can do it."

6. **Avoiding the "Cues."** It was noted earlier in this chapter that there are "cue-induced" cravings (another form of triggers). These cues become associated with drinking, such as a football game on TV, playing the guitar before going to the bar, driving past a tavern on the way home from work, or a birthday party. The result is that once the cue is present, then the alcoholic experiences cravings for a drink. Initially, the person is best advised to stay away from the cues—drive a different way home, not watch football on TV, and put the guitar away for a while. Later on, when the cravings diminish, these cues may be reintroduced into the person's lifestyle with appropriate adjustments to ensure they do not set off the cravings again.

7. Planned Escapes. Similar to the need to avoid certain cues, there will be times when it is prudent or necessary for the alcoholic to escape or simply leave situations. For example, there may be a late afternoon work meeting and when the meeting is finished it is customary to sit around and have a few drinks. In these cases the alcoholic needs to leave and say something like, "Look I have to head home now." Similarly, when the spur of the moment or surprise situations arise where alcohol is present, such as a chance meeting with friends who are drinking, it is simplest for the alcoholic to politely take leave and not have to deal with the cravings that will inevitably arise.

There are two central thoughts on cravings highlighted in Box 5.1.

BOX 5.1: Key Thoughts on Cravings

- The cravings will *subside* over time if the person does not yield to them.

- If the person does yield, and takes alcohol, then the cravings are substantially *strengthened* and will become more intense and persistent next time.

Checklist and Action Plan for Cravings

The following checklist and action plan is solely intended as a guide for alcoholics who have begun, or are about to begin, the challenging task of quitting drinking. While an individual may have other ways of addressing cravings than what is described in this book, the strong stance we take is that the individual must have a plan, which ideally, is developed with a support person. If not this plan, then another plan needs to be formulated. Cravings are too powerful and too persistent to be contested without a solid plan that is consistently followed. Moreover, when the cravings strike, it is particularly important to have responses at the ready. For most, especially initially, the cravings are very strong and it is hard to think or decide what to do. So by having thought through a plan, one is ready to respond, which will help in overcoming these cravings with less difficulty.

In the development of this checklist and action plan to address cravings, items are taken from the content of this chapter and listed in the *Items* column of the checklist. The top portion is for recording when and where cravings occur. Recovering alcoholics select which items might best work for them in the *Yes/No* column, in the second portion of the checklist, and then they provide a brief description of how they intend to use the item in the *Notes* column. The action plan section is used to list additional thoughts or steps needed to implement the items selected.

Note: Some individuals have found it helpful to make a small copy of this form and carry it around with them in their wallet or purse to remind them to track the cravings and what they do about them and to note their responses.

A blank form for the checklist Appendix C: Form 5.1, Checklist and Action Plan for Cravings, is presented in the appendices section and an example is described in Illustration 5.1.

Background: Beil, a 22-year-old house painter, is in his 2nd month of abstinence and has gone to talk to a friend who has several years of sobriety. Beil wanted to talk about his cravings. Beil stated, "I don't know when they are going to hit. It seems like they are going on all day long or always just around the corner." His friend suggested filling out the following form and following the suggestions for addressing cravings from this chapter. Beil agreed saying that he is determined to quit drinking forever but would like to get some help with these cravings. Beil has an iPhone and works on developing websites from his home evenings.

ILLUSTRATION 5.1: Checklist and Action Plan for Cravings

DESCRIPTION OF CRAVINGS

Measurement	Response	Notes
1. Frequency (How often?)	*Every day late afternoon*	*We get together after work around 5 pm for a drink. I drink sodas but I sure feel like a beer. Even when we don't get together I still get the craving for a beer at this time every day.*
2. Duration (How long?)	*Varies, usually about two hours sometimes longer but never less than two hours*	*The craving is always strongest around 5:00 which is the time we get together. Then it tapers off some but is still there sometimes for up to 2 hours and begins anytime in the afternoon.*
3. Intensity (How strong?)	*Very strong around five then tapers off but does not go away*	*The craving is strongest when the guys are ordering and even when I am by myself it is strongest around 5 pm. I get the jits and feel very restless. Later on it subsides and then I just feel like having a drink. I feel the taste*

ILLUSTRATION 5.1: *Continued*

STRATEGIES TO DEFUSE CRAVINGS

Tools	Does this Tool Apply to Me?		Notes
Having the Right Mindset			
1. Knowing what to expect	<u>Yes</u>	No	*I have my symptoms written out and on my iPhone in a pdf file. I read them before 5 pm. Not sure if this helps or makes it worse.*
2 It will get worse before it gets better	<u>Yes</u>	No	*I have been told this but it is hard to get it into my brain when the cravings are there.*
3. Expect uncertainty between cravings	Yes	<u>No</u>	*Not really a problem. I just keep busy at work and the cravings come and go.*
4. It too shall pass	<u>Yes</u>	No	*I keep telling myself this and have a recording on my iPhone I play at times.*
5. View cravings as enticements	Yes	<u>No</u>	*I see it more as pressure and I have to be firm and resist.*
6. Realize cravings are irrational	<u>Yes</u>	No	*Yes, I understand this, but the battle goes on.*
Procedures for Defusing Cravings			
1. Contact a friend	<u>Yes</u>	No	*Yes, I need to do more of this. That is why I came to see you.*
2. Get busy	<u>Yes</u>	No	*When I get antsy being busy is the only thing that works for me.*
3. Use relaxation strategies	Yes	<u>No</u>	*This does not work for me. I am too antsy but surfing on the net with my iPhone helps.*
4. Use symbols	<u>Yes</u>	No	*My iPhone is my lifeline. I have this running hot when the cravings are strong.*
5. Think it through	Yes	<u>No</u>	*Thinking is tough for me in the heat of the cravings. Later on I think about how I must never yield to the cravings.*
6. Avoid the "cues"	<u>Yes</u>	No	*At first I thought it best to not gather with my buddies after work. But they're my friends. However, I decided I wouldn't stick around too long especially when they're getting loaded. I just take off now after a bit.*
7. Planned escapes	<u>Yes</u>	No	*I got them to expect me to take off after a little bit as they knew I work developing websites at home—kinda moonlighting.*

ILLUSTRATION 5.1: *Continued*

ACTION PLAN

- *I decided to meet with my friend more and talk about cravings and how to manage them.*

- *My iPhone is the key. I really need to keep that in my hand and run it hot when I know the cravings are coming and when they are there.*

- *I can visit with by buddies after work for a short time and then make sure I take off and go home and work on developing the websites which not only helps my income but also occupies my mind.*

- *I plan to keep the website development going at home especially after work when cravings are strongest.*

Chapter Summary

Cravings, the powerful urges to drink alcohol, play a critical role in maintaining alcoholism and must be systematically addressed when a person decides to quit alcohol use and gain lifelong sobriety. Once the person makes a commitment to become sober, planning for management of the cravings has to occur as an essential component of his or her intervention.

The first step is for the individual to be fully informed on what cravings are and how they operate. Initially, alcoholics turn to alcohol to gain respite from certain needs that are not being met in other ways. However, alcoholics begin to drink more often and drink greater quantities. A point is reached where they become dependent on alcohol. Alcohol becomes the need in itself and the body begins to crave alcohol. The body then becomes highly agitated until these cravings are only assuaged by consuming alcohol.

Strategies are presented to assist individuals in managing the cravings when they arise based on having the right mindset and using specific procedures for shifting the focus from cravings to other thoughts and activities. The role of a support person is also highlighted to help the recovering alcoholic through this difficult period. Above all, recovering alcoholics must *not yield* to the cravings, otherwise it will be that much harder to control them next time around. The message presented is that while cravings provide considerable discomfort to the individual and can be quite persistent, they will subside if the individual persists with common practices and seeks support as needed.

Tools for Meeting Initial Needs

6

We use all kinds of ways to escape – all addictions stem from this moment when we meet our edge and we just can't stand it. We feel we have to soften it, pad it with something, and we become addicted to whatever it is that seems to ease the pain.

— Pema Chodron

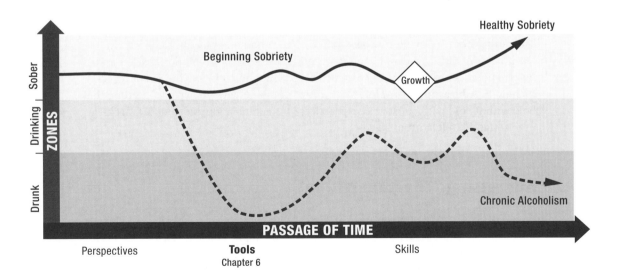

Thy he recovering alcoholic's journey is now at a crossroad. One pathway leads to alcoholism which has, until now, been well worn by the individual. The other pathway leads to sobriety. By undertaking these initial two interventions, quitting alcohol (Chapter 4, Detoxification) and resisting cravings (Chapter 5, Defusing Cravings) the individual has made giant strides in making a choice for the sobriety path. It is as if a red stop-light appears at the entrance of the path to alcoholism with the individual emphatically saying, "I am not going that way!" A green light appears at the entrance of the pathway to sobriety which must now be the pathway of choice. Figure 6.1: Tools for Meeting Initial Needs illustrates this juncture.

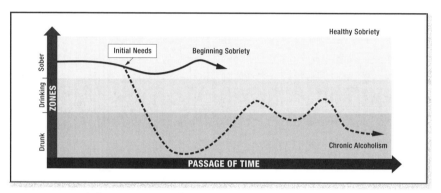

FIGURE 6.1: Tools for Meeting Initial Needs

The purpose of this chapter is to explain the next challenges facing alcoholics in the process of quitting alcohol and to describe the details for rebuilding skills and helpful practices for embarking on this new pathway to sobriety. The major topics include: 1. Addressing "The Hole Within," 2. Knowing what to expect, 3. Filling the hole within void with constructive practices, 4. Keeping a journal, and 5. Checklist and Action Plan for Initial Needs.

Addressing "The Hole Within"

To break up the cycle of alcoholism and create a new pathway to sobriety, the first major intervention is to quit drinking period (Chapter 4, Tools for Detoxification). The second intervention is to manage the cravings, (Chapter 5, Tools for Defusing Cravings). At this stage the individual has quit drinking and has addressed the cravings, it is only a matter of time before the original needs and new needs will surface. The initial needs, such as feelings of loneliness, stress, or the need to have fun with other drinkers, will re-emerge as if with a vengeance. Alcoholics become dependent on alcohol to meet these needs, and if relief is delayed, the individual experiences increasing discomfort, anxiety, and pain—they begin to experience *the hole within*. Essentially, alcohol was used as a tool to help the individual *address* these needs, so once the person quits alcohol, it can be expected that the needs will return. This is because whatever the reasons were for creating the needs, the needs were never addressed. The recourse the individual chose was to drink alcohol which resulted in relief from the problems or needs. *No skills were learned to address the needs.* The only remedy was to use alcohol to mask the problems. Consequently, when the person quits alcohol the same problems and needs will return.

Moreover, new needs not previously experienced typically emerge because the individual is suddenly in a new space– sober. Now the person is particularly vulnerable because these emerging needs with accompanying intense feelings, such as pain, anxiety, fear, boredom, or discomfort, are present. In addition, the individuals will be in situations that are relatively new for them such as managing their home, their job, or dealing with relationships. Since the old remedy of using alcohol is not an option, there is a significant *void* present—they experience the hole within. The person, for example, may experience stress but cannot drink for relief; the person feels lonely but cannot go to a bar for company and begin drinking; the person wants to have a good time but cannot go on a drinking binge; the person has trouble sleeping because he or she has been using alcohol to get to sleep; or the person feels a strange lack of focus and indecisiveness as a result of being free of alcohol. In effect, needs are present in force but the individual has been disarmed by removing the alcohol option. So how is this hole within to be managed? The solution lies in creating a new pathway that involves developing a new set of skills to address these previously unmet and emerging new needs in productive and sensible ways.

Knowing What to Expect

One of the most important steps for alcoholics when they begin to forge a pathway to sobriety is to understand what they are up against before they begin the process. A useful analogy is to consider the plight of a person who has to undergo major surgery. Typically, this person is informed by medical staff of what the procedure involves, the pain it may cause, the many restrictions following the surgery, and all the possible side effects. This information can be quite daunting for many patients.

However, the choices are clear. Does the patient want to *endure* all this for the short term and go on to *enjoy* a reasonable quality of life? Or, does the patient want to allow the medical condition to slowly (or quickly) consume the person's life with suffering and possibly death? Most people opt for the surgery and tough out the initial suffering and limitations.

A similar decision applies to alcoholics. Is the alcoholic willing to endure the initial suffering, hardships, and emptiness (the hole within) in order to have a healthy lifestyle free of the harmful and life-threatening effects of excessive alcohol use? However, before this decision is made, the alcoholic needs to be fully informed of the challenges that will arise from quitting alcohol, particularly in regard to finding new ways to meet previously unmet and newly emerging needs. In this way the alcoholics are more likely to be successful in their decision to quit alcohol, avoid a relapse, endure the initial hardships, and establish a new pathway to sobriety.

The extent of the difficulties facing the alcoholic will depend on the stage of alcoholism reached Level I, Tremors; Level II, Hallucinations and Seizures; or Level III, Delirium Tremens (see Chapter 4). Individuals who have reached Level III, Delirium Tremens can expect more problems than those who have reached Level I, Tremors.

It is strongly recommended that a professional, a sponsor, or an informed friend explain to the alcoholic what is likely to be in store and provide the necessary encouragement and support to help the alcoholic get through this stage of recovery.

The Need for Stop-Gap Measures

The long-term plan for the alcoholic is to embark on a new pathway to sobriety designed to meet his or her needs leading to a healthy sober lifestyle (detailed in Section Three). However, once the person has quit drinking, the individual will be confronted with many needs that can prove to be overwhelming and discouraging unless immediate steps are taken. These steps are simply *stop-gap* measures to help the person get through this initial period. It is analogous to "let's stop the bleeding first." The primary purpose of these initial steps is to help the alcoholic assume some level of stability or some level of homeostasis following withdrawal from alcohol. Once such a level of equilibrium has been attained, the alcoholic is in a position to undertake more systematic, individual, and long-term skill-building measures (presented in Section Three).

While there is quite an array of stop-gap activities and interventions an individual may use, it is recommended that the choices meet the following criteria:

1. Can be readily or immediately accessed

2. Has the capacity to take up a considerable amount of time

3. Is basically constructive versus something that is harmful or questionable

4. Has some evidence of effectiveness based on successful use by other recovering alcoholics

5. Is affordable

6. Can be accomplished individually or with others (without causing dependence)

7. Is within the skill range of the individual (not something the person may struggle with thereby adding to the problems)

Identifying and Managing the Foremost Emerging Needs

Human needs have been a rich subject of study for many decades and several models have emerged in the literature over the years such as Maslow's hierarchy of needs, Herzberg's two-factor theory of motivation, Alderfer's ERG model, and others. (See Box 6.1 for a list of resources.) Rosenfeld, Culbertson, and Magnusson (1992) in an extensive review of major theories of human needs concluded that no single theory can adequately account for the full range of human needs, motivation, wants, and behaviors.

However, one factor is common among these various theories and models; there is some kind of hierarchy or progression between human needs. Hertnon (2005) described a simplified hierarchical model in terms of two basic progressive needs, *survival* and *betterment*. The more basic level, survival needs, relate to physical and mental well-being. The next level, betterment needs, refers to higher needs such as respect from others, self reliance, and self-esteem. Meeting survival needs are considered to be a *prerequisite* to meeting the second need, betterment.

This chapter covers tools for immediate survival needs related to emerging needs and filling the hole within with constructive practices. The second order of needs, skills for betterment, will be presented in Section Three: Skills for Healthy Sobriety. In terms of the new pathway to sobriety, *survival* needs refer to steps at the beginning of the pathway, while *betterment* needs apply to steps further along the pathway.

Some of the major basic survival needs likely to emerge during this intervention stage of initial recovery are: filling the hole within with constructive practices, taking care of one's physical well-being, establishing support, dealing with loneliness, living with diminished life skills, dealing with pressure to drink at social occasions, avoiding the trouble spots, and managing alcohol rituals.

Each of these needs will be briefly described along with established tools for meeting these needs.

BOX 6.1: Resources for Theories on Human Needs

Alderfer, C. P. (1972). *Existence, relatedness, and Growth: Human Needs in Organizational Settings.* Glencoe, IL: Free Press

Dean, H. (2010). *Understanding Human Need.* Bristol, UK: Policy Press.

Hertnon, S. (2005). *Theory of Universal Human Needs.* Auckland, NZ: Nakedize Publishing.

Herzberg, F. (1959). *The Motivation to Work.* New York: John Wiley and Sons.

Maslow, A. (1954). *Motivation and Personality.* New York: Harper and Row.

Rosenfeld, P., Culbertson, A. L., & Magnusson, P. (1992). *Human Needs: A Literature Review and Cognitive Life Span Model.* Report presented to the Navy Personnel Research and Development Center, San Diego, CA.

Living with Diminished Life Skills

Recovering alcoholics often find they are at a loss to deal with the most basic life skills such as doing their laundry; cleaning their room, apartment, or home; making a shopping list; or finding their way around the grocery store. Making concrete, practical decisions and problem solving become huge challenges, even to the point of a crisis, for them. They don't know where to start.

Two suggestions for managing these diminished life skills are: firstly to to understand that this problem is normal and to be expected and, second, seek help from a family member, friend, or a personal support person described in an upcoming section, Obtaining Personal Support.

Moreover, alcoholics in this early stage of recovery often experience mood swings of emotional highs and lows (not unlike the experiences of a person with the debilitating disability of manic-depression). During these periods the recovering alcoholic may become over-excited about something and make a reckless decision. For example, individuals may feel so good being alcohol free– that they rush out and buy a new car or head to the mall and load up with new clothes, often the first clothes they see. Again, the best safeguard to help in controlling such impulsive decisions is to work closely with a support person.

Filling the Hole Within Void with Constructive Practices

Alcoholics experience a difficult and threatening void when they quit drinking. The reason is obvious and to be expected. For some time, alcohol consumption has been *a way of life* for them (for many years in most cases). If they are not drinking, they are hung over or making moves to resume drinking. Now that they quit, what is the immediate effect? They come face to face with a consuming void or hole within. As a recovering alcoholic so aptly shared at a meeting:

> "The great part about sobriety is that you can feel again. The lousy
> part of sobriety is that you can feel again."

The challenge is to manage these powerful feelings in effective ways and set the stage for enjoying sobriety with an enhanced quality of life. To accomplish this, the alcoholic must find *constructive* ways to fill this void. The word *constructive* is critical because some alcoholics turn to practices that may fill the void but are harmful, such as excessive gambling, sexually acting out, overeating, spending binges, drugs, and crime. Constructive practices fill the void by helping the individual to *remain sober* as well as build a *reasonable quality of life* (a major theme of this chapter).

Common tools to use in productive ways when quitting alcohol:

- Exercise by taking walks, going to the gym, or working out at home

- Gardening or yard work

- Routine house cleaning

- Hobbies, home projects, personal projects

- Movies or theater performances

- Playing or listening to music

The remainder of this chapter provides information on other strategies for filling the void in constructive ways.

Taking Care of One's Physical Well-Being

One of the many harmful effects of alcoholism is its impact on the physical well-being of the individual. For example, the alcoholic neglects several areas of normal well-being such as a balanced diet, regular sleep, personal appearance, and, in some cases, personal hygiene (refer to Chapter 1 for fuller accounts of the harmful effects of alcoholism).   Shortly after a person quits alcohol, these personal areas of neglect usually become a serious concern and must be effectively addressed. Time and effort spent on improving personal well-being is time and effort spent constructively filling the voids.

> **Sleep.** Alcoholics, as a rule, have no trouble sleeping. They simply black out or pass out. However, the recovering alcoholic has to learn a *new way* to go to sleep now without resorting to alcohol-induced sleep. Strategies commonly used by recovering alcoholics to bring on sleep include:
>
> - physical exercise prior to sleeping
> - reading, TV, and movies

- use of relaxation practices such as yoga-type exercises, controlled breathing, and recorded relaxation music and sounds

- over-the-counter sleeping pills.

Note: The recovering alcoholic is strongly encouraged to see a doctor if persistent sleeping problems arise. Under no circumstances should narcotics be employed otherwise a new and equally, if not more, harmful addiction will be developed. Avoid at all costs replacing one chemical dependency (alcohol) with another (narcotics and overuse of prescription sleeping pills).

Diet. Alcoholics do not eat well in general. They eat what they can get their hands on without much thought to what they are eating. The recovering alcoholic needs to establish new and certainly better eating habits. One recovering alcoholic reported:

"I don't eat much these days. It seems my metabolism has changed when the booze was taken away. It's like a baby that's been weaned I suppose."

Plan a weekly menu. One of the surest ways to control or shape eating habits is to plan a menu for the day or the week. In this way the person is likely to eat a balanced diet and stay within the budget.

Eat healthy food three times a day. However, some alcoholics may be unable to plan menus initially. In these cases, the alcoholics should try to eat three times a day and choose food that has nutritional value. Time that was spent destructively seeking and consuming alcohol can now be spent constructively seeking and consuming healthy foods.

Drink lots of water. The recovering alcoholic is encouraged to drink reasonably large volumes of water throughout the day. A common practice is to drink a minimum of three large glasses a day (one in the morning, one in the afternoon, and one in the evening). This healthy practice helps the individuals to quench their thirst but also gives them something to have in their hand and, most importantly, helps to cleanse their system of the toxins caused by alcohol.

Personal Hygiene. The recovering alcoholic usually needs to establish, or re-establish, hygiene routines:

- showering or bathing

- brushing and flossing dental hygiene

- doing laundry on a regular basis

- grooming, haircuts and attire.

Establishing Support and Dealing with Loneliness

The feeling of loneliness is often quite acute when a person quits alcohol. These individuals have been in regular contact with others who drink and now drinking is out of the question; they find themselves alone.

Here are two time-tested keys to addressing loneliness and to filling this void constructively:

1. Join a support group

2. Work with a personal support person

Joining a Support Group

Connecting with others through participation in support groups is a well documented and widely used strategy for meeting needs of people. There are many diverse groups for individuals who share a common and often debilitating affliction, for example, sufferers of diabetes, cancer survivors, veterans of wars, weight watchers, and abused women. These support groups are helpful because those who attend are made to feel welcome *immediately*. The only prerequisite seems to be that individuals have suffered, want to do better, want to help each other, and want to be with kindred people.

There are many nationally known and readily accessible groups that provide support to recovering alcoholics. In addition, there are groups designed to serve multiple addictions such as combinations of alcoholism, gambling, and narcotics.

The key is for alcoholics to find the right match for their needs. Some of these support groups include the following:

- Alcoholics Anonymous, AA (www.aa.org)

- Narcotics Anonymous, NA (www.na.org)

- Gamblers Anonymous, GA (www.recovery-world.com/Gamblers-Anonymous.html)

- Smart Recovery (www.smartrecovery.org)

- Secular Organization for Sobriety, SOS (www.cfiwest.org/sos/index.htm)

- Women for Sobriety, WFS (www.womenforsobriety.org)

- Life Ring (www.lifering.org)

- 16 Steps for Discovery and Empowerment (http://mixedbag.us/16steps.htm)

Recovering alcoholics are strongly encouraged to find a support group compatible with their needs and *attend the meetings.* By regular attendance at the meetings, alcoholics are provided fellowship, acceptance, and encouragement. The structure of the meetings typically affords nonjudgmental assistance, accountability, reminders, and many useful suggestions. In addition, the recovering alcoholic is given the opportunity to make new friends, participate in functions as desired, have access to an array of services as needed, and can receive support at many basic daily living skills such as such as help in moving, setting up their living conditions, and in obtaining essentials (food, furniture, clothing, toiletries, and cleaning gear).

Obtaining Personal Support

In addition to the fellowship and friendship that support groups provide, recovering alcoholics usually need help and support at a *personal* level. In many cases the recovering alcoholic might be like Humpty-Dumpty who "fell off the wall"– they are broken people who struggle to put themselves together. However, unlike Humpty-Dumpty, they can be "put together again." Recovering alcoholics typically need help to unravel what it is that drove them to excessive alcohol use in the first place and to start over again on a new path to sobriety. What are their needs? How do these needs manifest themselves? In what other ways can these needs be met? One of the time-tested strategies for helping a recovering alcoholic at this level is *one-on-one assistance* such as a:

- sponsor from one of the various support groups listed in the previous section

- counselor

- therapist (individual and small group)

- member of the clergy or pastoral care provider from a religious group

- close friend who has been in recovery for some time

Key to Success

The authors cannot stress enough that two of the most important construc-tive strategies for success-fully undertaking the pathway to sobriety are:

- Regular support group attendance.

- Obtaining a personal support person (such as a sponsor).

The support person must be involved with potentially reckless decisions, such as buying a brand new car or a whole new wardrobe. There has to be an understanding that the advice of the support person will be listened to, especially when it is in opposition to what the individual wants.

Dealing with the Pressures to Drink

While it is a huge challenge for the alcoholic to quit drinking, another aspect of that challenge is dealing with all the pressures to drink that arise from other people and social situations which include the former drinking locations, "drinking buddies," parties, special celebrations, and dinners.

> **Drinking Locations.** If a recovering alcoholic had a standard practice of drinking at certain locations, then it is especially important for the alcoholic to avoid those places.
>
> > *Avoid places of temptation.* Someone may say, "Come on by and see us. We have plenty of nonalcoholic drinks." The issue is why would you put yourself under that kind of pressure? It is very difficult for a recovering alcoholic, especially in the early stages of recovery, to stand around drinking sodas or nonalcoholic drinks watching the

others drink alcohol, having to explain why you are not drinking if it comes up, and having to listen to the endless laughter and repetitive stories after people have been drinking for a while. It is wiser just to avoid these places and try to seek constructive alternatives (the personal support person usually can provide helpful options).

Meet for coffee or lunch. Some alcoholics have reported that when they approach certain gatherings or locations where drinking is underway, they break out into a sweat, get the shakes, and feel panic. There is no loss of face here in making a U-turn, leaving and going somewhere else. It is very important for alcoholics to listen to and take action when their body reacts to certain events or situations.

"Drinking Buddies." The recovering alcoholic will surely run into situations where former drinking friends will say, "You can still come see us. We'd like to see you." Again you will run into the same difficulties of being the odd one out. They are drinking: you are not. Some recovering alcoholics suggest something like, "Yes. I'd like to see you. Could we have coffee or lunch?" If the answer is basically a flat no, then you know where you stand. Your presence is just part of the package of drinking. However, if the person is willing to have lunch or coffee, then you know that person really wants to see you and stay in touch even though you are not drinking.

Some individuals recovering from late stage alcoholism may have very limited social opportunities. For example, they may gather with their buddies under the bridge, in alleys, or other out-of-the-way locations. These individuals must avoid these settings and try to find other gatherings such as the mission or church support services.

Parties and Gatherings. There is no question, parties and gatherings are tough to manage with everyone milling around drinking while the recovering alcoholic is struggling to "be normal" and have a good time without drinking. Real tension is experienced and pressure is certainly there to drink. The recovering alcoholics sense that "everyone notices" that they are not drinking now which leads to some discomfort from being different and perhaps from feeling pressure to explain themselves.

Moreover, there is the ongoing pressure to take a drink. The host may be passing out drinks, a friend may say, "Who needs a drink?" or "Can I get you a drink?" and so it goes. One helpful suggestion is for the recovering alcoholics to get a nonalcoholic drink in their hand as soon as possible. In this way, when they are seen to be holding a drink, they are less likely to be asked if they need a drink or to be offered a drink.

Some individuals find it helps to hang out with those who are not drinking alcohol. More and more people are refraining from drinking alcohol, some are designated drivers, some are on medication, others are trying to be moderate and not drink on this occasion.

Keeping a cell phone in hand allows instant phone calls or texting to a support person. Also holding a phone in the hand or a nonalcoholic drink can help prevent others from offering an alcoholic drink.

Another important strategy that helps to reduce pressure to drink is to *minimize time spent* at these gatherings. A common practice is to arrive somewhat late and to leave early. For some events it is customary to have a few drinks before things get underway. In these cases it is better for the alcoholic to come later and avoid this time set for drinking.

Recovering alcoholics have to keep reminding themselves that it is *their decision to quit alcohol* and theirs only. They do not have to explain themselves to anyone and they certainly do not have to convince anyone of their decision. This mindset is difficult to attain but needs to be worked at constantly.

Avoiding the Trouble Spots

Recovering alcoholics are well aware of routines where they are most likely to drink. These routines must be changed. If an individual has the practice of dropping into a certain bar on the way home, then he or she must go somewhere else at this time. If a little gathering occurs at the end of the day to have a few drinks, then recovering alcoholics must excuse themselves from such gatherings and run errands or do something else. Some recovering alcoholics have had rituals or habits of having a night cap or after-dinner drink or before-dinner drink. These practices must stop. Some recovering alcoholics try substituting another drink on these occasions. This is difficult to accomplish because all of the triggers are there to drink alcohol. It is far simpler to abandon the routine entirely and do something entirely different such as answer email or do a crossword puzzle or walk the dog. The critical step is to identify these routines and change them in a constructive way.

Managing Alcohol Rituals

There are many festive occasions where it is customary to drink alcohol. For example, there is the ritual of using champagne to toast someone for graduating, getting married, securing a new job or promotion, having a baby, someone turning 100 years old, and to greet the new year. It is very easy to grab a champagne glass in the excitement of the moment or even pressure of the moment, to make the toast. The drinking is quite secondary to making the toast. On these occasions it is best to have a glass of some nonalcoholic drink in your hand already. It may be helpful to realize that the occasion is what is being celebrated and whether alcohol is used or not is really irrelevant or at most secondary to the event.

Keeping a Journal

There is no question that the recovering alcoholics will experience a range of emotions, thoughts, and challenges during their early days of sobriety. Tracking these experiences has proven to be very helpful to some individuals. The whole point is that whatever is going on needs to be *processed* by the individuals otherwise they may become confused, discouraged, and more than likely to begin drinking again.

This processing is best accomplished through regular visits with a personal support person such as a sponsor or counselor (see earlier section in this chapter, Obtaining Personal Support). However, some individuals are capable of processing the early recovering period by themselves. The key issue is that the processing and reflection needs to occur.

Many recovering alcoholics have found it very helpful to keep a daily journal for this purpose. It is understood that some individuals may not be capable at this stage of maintaining a journal for any number of reasons. However, there are decided advantages in keeping a journal if at all possible. One individual commented that when he kept a journal he realized that he had been drinking to escape from himself. By writing things down he learned much about himself, which at first he did not like, but as time passed he was able to sort it out and become comfortable with himself and his life.

Journal entries provide a focus for what the individual may be experiencing and also provide the basis for reflection and processing, either by oneself or with a personal support person (such as a sponsor). Topics that are typically included in a journal are listed below followed by an example of a journal entry in Box 6.2.

Journal Topics

- Major feelings such as anger, sadness, loneliness, pleasure

- Cravings and how they were dealt with

- Decisions and choices (good ones and poor ones)

- Drawings or doodles that may have some meaning

- Telling thoughts and insights

- Something said or written (quotes, phrases)

- Reflections

- Nagging thoughts or feelings

BOX 6.2: Example of Journal Entry

Date: June 12

Coffee with the Wednesday Group

Lana said that she was tired of having the same relationship with different people. Really hit home … I always pick the needy ones … and drink to escape … Everything I do though seems at times to just be collecting the reasons to drink. I guess I drank because that is what I do. I really like the Sunshine group … My sponsor has been nagging to get a group … I think I will pick this one … good guys … I feel comfortable … Yep that is what I will do.

Checklist and Action Plan for Initial Needs

The following checklist and action plan is intended as a guide for recovering alcoholics to help them address the unmet needs and emerging needs that set the occasion for their drinking. It is assumed these needs will emerge as a matter of course and that the individual should have a plan to manage them in constructive ways.

This checklist and action plan to address the unmet and emerging needs. Items are taken from the content of this chapter and listed in the *Item* column of the checklist. Readers are directed to select which items might best work for them in the *Yes /No* column and then provide a brief description in the *Notes* column of how they intend to use the item. The list is by no means exhaustive, so recovering alcoholics are encouraged to add items that are important to them under the heading *Other* and in the Action Plan section to list additional thoughts or steps needed to implement the items selected.

A blank form for this checklist and action plan is presented in the appendices section, Appendix D: Form 6.1, Checklist and Action Plan for Initial Needs, and an example is described in Illustration 6.1.

Background: Barbara is 45 and a single divorced mom. Her ex-husband divorced her because of her drinking. She was able to keep custody of her child because of her sister's involvement and the husband's job took him out of town a lot. She had been active with sports but her drinking took all her time. She decided to address her problem and went to detox treatment and became involved with a sponsor. Presently she is supported by alimony.

ILLUSTRATION 6.1: Checklist and Action Plan for Initial Needs

Item	Selection (Underline)		Notes
Preparing Oneself Beforehand	<u>Yes</u>	No	*I made a plan last week with my sponsor and it scares me but I am determined to go for it. Not sure what lies ahead really.*
Filling the Void with Constructive Practices	<u>Yes</u>	No	*I am going to spend as much time getting sober as I did getting drunk. I will go to my AA meetings and in my spare time I will volunteer more time with the soccer club.*
Taking Care of One's Physical-Well Being	<u>Yes</u>	No	*I understand that it will take time before I can sleep regularly. I'll see how I do or use some sleeping pills if need be.*
Sleep	<u>Yes</u>	No	
Diet	Yes	<u>No</u>	*I'll get help with planning a healthy menu and buying groceries within my budget AND cut way back on fast foods. I also need to restock my kitchen as I have let all of that slide.*
Personal Hygiene and Appearance	<u>Yes</u>	No	
Living with Diminished Life Skills	<u>Yes</u>	No	*I have let a lot of things go and now have to start again. I have to spend more time with my child and be more consistent. I have to organize myself for cooking meals, keeping the house clean, doing my job with the soccer club and volunteer work.* *Also, the house is a mess so I need to get it cleaned up and organized again. My sister will help me. At least I haven't let my appearance slide.*
Establishing Support			*I go to meetings twice a week– Women for Sobriety (WFS) and once a week to AA. I also get support from the soccer moms*
Support Groups —Meetings	<u>Yes</u>	No	
Personal Support	<u>Yes</u>	No	*Following detox I chose a sponsor and we meet regularly and I call her often. I get together with my sister twice a week.*

ILLUSTRATION 6.1 *Continued*

Dealing with the Pressures to Drink	<u>Yes</u>	No	*I'll stop going to bridge group as they drink during the game. I will avoid the soccer mom parties or just go with the moms who don't*
Drinking Locations	<u>Yes</u>	No	*drink. I will gather with people who do not drink. My sponsor and sister are helping me find*
"Drinking Buddies"	<u>Yes</u>	No	*gatherings that are alcohol free.*
Parties and Gatherings	<u>Yes</u>	No	*I was at a birthday party and there was a toast and I made sure I had a glass of apple cider in my hand instead of champagne and I kept my cell phone handy and texted my sponsor.*
Avoiding the Trouble Spots	<u>Yes</u>	No	*I don't visit after soccer with parents who drink. I now head off to do grocery shopping or begin dinner preparation. I will examine my routines and change all the ones that involve alcohol.*
Managing Alcohol Rituals	<u>Yes</u>	No	*I am a little overweight and I used to jog so I will pick up jogging again.*
Keeping a Journal	<u>Yes</u>	No	*I have a notebook but I just have trouble staying with it for more than a sentence or two. My sponsor understands my difficulty and just encourages me to do what I can when I can.*
Other	Yes	No	

ACTION PLAN

The main parts of my action plan to begin with are:

- *Attend meetings (WFS and AA) twice a week (Not sure yet which group works best for me).*

- *Get help from my sister with reorganizing the house and developing menus immediately.*

- *Strongly avoid any of the places, times, or groups where I have been drinking.*

- *Schedule volunteer work at the Al-Anon second-hand store and with the soccer club.*

- *Get fitness plans for myself beginning with walking and building up to jogging with some of the moms (after children have been taken to school and before the noon meeting).*

- *Spend time with child after dinner—playing games, helping with homework, going to store, reading, watching TV.*

- *Make phone calls to make contact with others after child is in bed.*

- *Begin to look for and think about possible part-time work.*

Chapter Summary

When alcoholics quit drinking it is not long before they come face to face with the very reasons that led them to become addicted to alcohol use in the first place, which have been identified as unmet needs. Not only that, the alcoholic will experience, quite quickly, a new set of needs, emerging needs, that can become quite overwhelming unless concrete steps are taken. Typically, most alcoholics establish patterns of drinking to excess because the alcohol enables them to meet certain needs, or repress them, such as to escape from stress or to relax and have a good time. But it is not long before the alcohol itself becomes the reason for drinking and these unmet needs become secondary concerns or are simply repressed. However, when the person quits drinking, these needs will re-emerge and become quite challenging. The recovering alcoholic not only has to deal with these formerly repressed needs but, in addition, will have to deal with the needs that arise from being newly sober after being alcohol dependent for an extended period.

This chapter focused on identifying the foremost needs likely to be encountered in these early stages of recovery and describing best-practice constructive strategies for managing them. A common thread with interventions for addressing these emerging needs following the cessation of drinking is to use stop gap measures to "grab anything that works" (given it is acceptable or constructive) so as to get through this challenging and daunting period. By so doing, the recovering alcoholic will be launching a new pathway, a beginning pathway to healthy sobriety. Two key support strategies were strongly recommended: first, regular participation in a support group; and second, regular access to a support person such as a sponsor. A checklist and action plan form was presented to enable individuals to examine their own situation and plan accordingly.

It is very important to understand that the recovering alcoholic's quest to manage these needs in constructive ways different from using alcohol, is *ongoing*. The focus in this chapter is restricted to assisting recovering alcoholics constructively manage the initial impact of quitting alcohol related to previously unmet and newly emerging needs. The goals have been to help the person through this challenging period, avoid any form of relapse, and set the stage for beginning a whole new pathway toward a sober and healthy lifestyle.

SECTION THREE

Skills for Healthy Sobriety

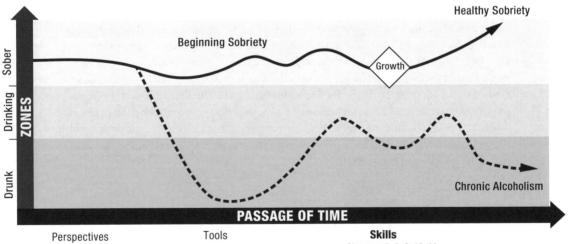

At this juncture the recovering alcoholic has made extraordinary gains— he or she has become sober. No one but the individual alcoholic knows the depths of the anguish and turmoil that has occurred to reach this point. It is indeed an accomplishment and every step and precaution should be taken to preserve the person's sobriety.

However, some recovering alcoholics, after a period of sobriety, may ask the question "Is there life after sobriety?" Or, more specifically, "What do I want life to be like after quitting alcohol?" The assumption is that just quitting drinking is not enough for them. Now the individual is ready for *betterment*. As one person said, "Quitting drinking makes my life *good*. Now I have to find out how to make it *better*." Or, in a similar vein, "Quitting drinking has made me a *better* person. Now I have to work on being the *best* person I can."

There is no assumption in these statements that the person is "cured of alcoholism" or has become overconfident and is highly likely to experience a relapse. Rather, some individuals may reach a point in their sobriety that their life has become dull or they still feel too dependent on others to sort out their problems as they arise or that they are still having mood swings that bother them.

Section Three is designed to respond fully to the core question "Can quality of life be enhanced after sobriety?" The section opens with Chapter 7: Key Considerations for Personal Growth, where a number of basic principles and cautions are addressed for enhancing recovering alcoholics' lifestyle. In the next four chapters, detailed descriptions of interventions are presented for helping the recovering alcoholic to learn skills in core human growth areas: Chapter 8: Skills for *Autonomous* Growth; Chapter 9: Skills for *Cognitive* Growth; Chapter 10: Skills for *Social* Growth; and Chapter 11: Skills for *Emotional* Growth. The diagram in the title page of this section shows interventions for these *skills* represented by the diamond labeled *Growth* on the pathway to healthy sobriety. Checklists and action plans with illustrations are presented for each of these personal growth areas (*autonomous, cognitive, social, and emotional*).

Key Considerations for Personal Growth

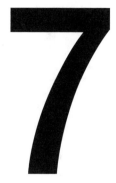

While stopping drinking is the necessary first step in recovery, it really only opens the door to the full experience of it.

— AA On-line Forum

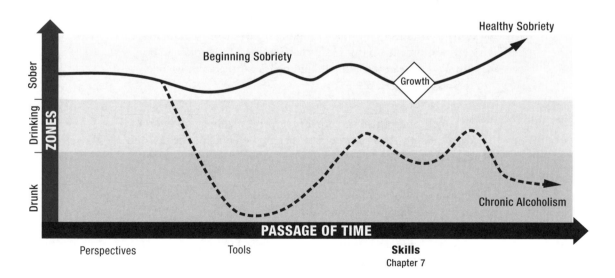

The following statements are about or made by individuals who have quit alcohol:

> "I have been sober for three years now and I am still very unhappy. It is very discouraging as I thought things would be better now that I have quit drinking."

> "Don't get me wrong. I am proud of my husband for getting sober. But seriously, he doesn't seem to be any different from when he was drinking. He lives in a dream world still, blames everybody all the time, and reacts mad to every silly little thing."

> "I don't get it. I have been sober for 14 years. I go to meetings 2–3 times a week, and for the most part I have always had a sponsor. But I still have mood swings and often feel very angry or depressed. I keep trying to find my demons but I don't get any relief—well not for long. I would give anything to find peace and calm but they elude me."

> "I am at the crossroads again. My choices are to start drinking again or live a life feeling miserable most of the time."

> "To be honest, I have given up on myself. I was rotten when I was drunk and feel very much afraid that I will drink again. My friends want me to do this or do that, but I feel too broken to do anything. I am safest staying in my shell regardless of how lonely or depressing it gets."

> "The only friends I have are other recovering alcoholics. I feel safe and accepted by them. It would be nice to 'step outside the box' but I am afraid to really."

> "It bugs me that when I was drinking I could put up with all sorts of things. Now that I have quit I find most things boring. Small talk with friends and family is real small now; I hate chatting on the phone and my job seems pretty pointless. Life seems to be just one dull day after another."

These statements ring true for many recovering alcoholics who make the herculean effort to quit drinking, work through the withdrawal symptoms from detoxification, struggle with and resist the cravings for alcohol, and stand firm when faced with the usual triggers and temptations to drink. Now they face an entirely different kind of hurdle and a formidable one at that—*the challenge of extending and expanding the quality of their lifestyle in addition to maintaining sobriety.*

In order to effectively address the factors involved in enhancing one's quality of life following sobriety, several key perspectives need to be considered, understood, and applied with due caution:

- This path is a choice not an expectation

- Know what to expect

- A skill-based approach

- Variability in problems experienced

- *Dry Drunk Syndrome*

- Understanding what is considered to be normal

- Don't throw out the baby with the bathwater

- Sobriety is an ongoing way of life

- Focus on the journey not the destination

- Quality of life is a result not a strategy in itself

- Emotional sobriety

- Four core elements of personal growth

- Pathway to healthy sobriety

This Path Is a Choice Not an Expectation

Some recovering alcoholics may be quite content to remain where they are, enjoying their sobriety and anchoring fully in the steps and support systems that enabled them to become sober. Others may want to systematically and carefully branch out into other areas to expand the quality of their lives. Information presented in these subsequent chapters is simply an *extension* to the life of sobriety. Some may wish to pursue this direction and others may not. The choice is there for the taking.

Know What to Expect

The old adage of "To be forewarned is to be forearmed" is especially true for recovering alcoholics. It is inevitable that when an alcoholic quits drinking a number of problems will be experienced related to basic life needs. Some individuals have problems related to social needs involving talking to people, getting along with others, and with facing fears they have not seen for years. For example, Bill, a recovering alcoholic, commented that he had been sober for a year and things were much better at home, but at gatherings he finds the conversations and small talk very boring and would prefer not to even be there. Murray, for example, worries that his friends will think less of him now that he has quit drinking, that he is a wimp, or that he cannot hold his drink.

The reason for the emergence of these kinds of fears related to daily living is that they have been repressed or masked through years of drinking. Now that the individual has quit alcohol these same needs and fears will surface as we discussed in Chapter 6, Tools for Meeting Initial Needs. The recommended measures were presented as *stop-gap* with the immediate goal of helping the person remain sober. Once the person remains sober for a period, it is only a matter of time before these needs re-emerge or other life-needs and experiences surface. It is important for the recovering alcoholic to understand that success in staying sober is *absolutely essential* but it is *not enough* when we are looking at quality of life factors. The person now has to systematically undertake additional steps on this pathway to achieve a *healthy* sobriety.

A Skill-Based Approach

A primary assumption in this book, and in this chapter, is that recovering alcoholics must learn a new set of skills to address their needs. In some cases the skills have never been learned and in others they have been buried because alcoholics spend most of their time drinking or dealing with the repercussions of drinking. If these skills are not learned and applied, then the alcoholic will have a lifelong sentence of discomfort or even misery and may resort to drinking alcohol again. Or, to a lesser degree, other alcoholics may spend their lives at a level of mediocrity and dissatisfaction. It is also crucial for the alcoholic to understand that these life skills have been thoroughly researched, well documented, and applied successfully across a very broad range of situations. Moreover, the skills have been widely applied with individuals in need of help and who are *not alcoholics*. Many individuals have a need to learn these skills for a host of reasons and the common approach is to break the skills down into simple, concrete, and understandable steps that can be taught and learned. Details of these skill-building procedures will be presented in Chapters 8–11 later in this section. These skills can be *learned* and they are quite *accessibl*e.

Variability in Problems Experienced

As expected there is a full range of experiences recovering alcoholics may encounter when they become sober. Some alcoholics will be challenged more seriously than others. For example, one individual may have to address boredom and intolerance of others while another may be confronted with deep-seated anger and depression. A major reason for this variability lies in the stage of alcoholism reached by the individual (see Chapter 4, *Tools for Detoxification)*. Individuals who have reached the highest stage, Stage III (DTs), can expect more serious problems after they quit drinking as they try to assimilate more fully into society than one, for example, who is at the *early stage* of alcoholism. Another key factor is the age of onset of the alcoholism. For example, individuals who become alcoholic in their teens and become sober in their early 30s can expect significant social problems because they did not learn these skills during this critical period in when they were younger. These alcoholics recovering from the late stage of alcoholism may need more support and have more limited goals, at least initially, when addressing life skills following sobriety than the individuals who began recovery at an earlier stage of alcoholism.

Dry Drunk Syndrome

A very helpful and insightful concept regarding the plight of recovering alcoholics, the *dry drunk syndrome*, was developed in the early literature of Alcoholics Anonymous (Solberg, 1983). This expression was coined to describe those individuals who had made the break and become sober ("dry") but still carried with them many of the behaviors so prevalent when they were drinking and drunk such as intolerance, regular outbursts of anger, blaming others, and very poor problem-solving skills. It is important to note that this condition is a steady or regular pattern of behavior as distinct from the typical ups and downs with moods many recovering alcoholics may experience. The following example listed in the opener to this chapter is a classic example of the dry drunk:

> Don't get me wrong. I am proud of my husband for getting sober. But seriously, he doesn't seem to be any different from when he was drinking. He lives in a dream world still, blames everybody all the time, and reacts mad to every silly little thing.

Some of the common behavioral descriptors for the dry drunk are listed in Box 7.1 (adapted from Solberg, 1983).

BOX 7.1: Common Behavioral Characteristics of the Dry Drunk

Grandiosity: Exaggerated or unrealistic expectations of one's abilities and importance.

Judgmentalism: Constantly being highly critical and negative toward others.

Intolerance: Reacts negatively and quickly to others' mistakes or differences.

Impulsivity: Acts without thinking and seeks immediate gratification of personal desires.

Indecisiveness: Cannot make up their mind, freezes or procrastinates at times of decision.

Manipulative: Pressures others and becomes very demanding to get what they want.

Self-Centered: Concerned with needs of self and often oblivious to others' feelings and needs.

Dishonest: Often lies, cheats, steals, and makes promises that are not fulfilled.

While many recovering alcoholics may not be considered to be *dry drunks,* more than likely they would possess some of these behavioral characteristics in varying degrees and would need to take steps to address them.

The dry drunk phenomenon is very strong information to recovering alcoholics and professionals in support service: quitting drinking alone is not sufficient to ensure that an individual will have a healthy and full life. Additional steps, the theme of this section (Chapters 7–11), need to be taken for the individual to attain a healthy and balanced lifestyle.

Dual Diagnoses. Some recovering alcoholics may encounter more persistent problems during sobriety as a function of a dual diagnoses or multiple diagnoses. For example, an individual who is contending with a *bipolar* mental health problem will have significant mood swings during new-found sobriety. The mental health disability confounds the problem and implies that the person needs help with managing the disability in conjunction with issues related to recovering from alcoholism.

Understanding What Is Considered to Be Normal

Recovering alcoholics can easily fall into the trap of putting themselves down and limiting their growth because they have an inflated and unrealistic perception of what is normal. Because normal people have been able to drink in moderation and have not experienced the weighty repercussions of excessive drinking and being drunk over a long period of time, they can be thought to have ongoing peace and serenity. This perception is far from reality. These so-called *normal people* also have their ups and downs personally, emotionally, mentally, and socially. They too have to constantly work at the skills needed for a healthy lifestyle. The recovering alcoholic must understand that emotional health and stability is something everyone has to invest in and work hard to attain. The need is common to all human beings. Moreover, the recovering alcoholic can learn from others, not only former alcoholics, how lifeskills can be developed and applied.

A similar perspective from what is normal can be gleaned from Joanne Greenberg's powerful novel of the '70s, *I Never Promised You a Rose Garden.* In this compelling story a skilled counselor was able to help a girl with schizophrenia to gradually let go of her fears and learn to live in the world even though the world was not necessarily that friendly or helpful. Again, it is crucial to understand that normal has its traps, imperfections, and problems. We do not live in a perfect world.

Don't Throw Out the Baby with the Bathwater

While the theme of this book is to help recovering alcoholics take whatever steps possible to develop and sustain a healthy lifestyle, a serious word of caution is needed. There is no question that recovering alcoholics are a vulnerable group of people. Some would say that they are a damaged group of people. Consequently, when they take steps to grow and become more tuned into a higher quality of life beyond just being sober, risk is involved. The individuals may take steps that do not work and may put them at risk for returning to drinking—experiencing a relapse. The individuals have made great strides to obtain sobriety, so it would be insensible to lose this sobriety, for example, by putting themselves at risk in their efforts to secure independence and social advancements.

We strongly recommend that recovering alcoholics use caution with their ongoing steps to grow and to maintain accessibility to their safety nets. The key is to take small measured steps so that if successful, then more steps can be taken. If unsuccessful, then controls are in place to protect the individuals and allow them to learn from the experience, not to get burned by it, and not to put their sobriety in jeopardy. Small, measured, incremental steps with adequate support are the key.

Sobriety is an Ongoing Way of Life

Just as life itself is composed of various stages of growth, so is a life of sobriety. The alcoholic begins with detoxification where the primary purpose is to quit drinking alcohol and to manage the effects of withdrawal. However, once the individual becomes successful in quitting alcohol, use other needs begin to surface. For example, the individual may be wholly dependent on others to maintain sobriety whether it be the support from fellowship or personal support. Some individuals may feel the need to take a bigger role in managing sobriety independently. That is they feel the need to become more self-reliant. Others may feel the need to expand their social network beyond family and the fellowship of alcohol support groups.

The key in each of these cases of expanded needs is to understand that a life of sobriety must be understood as a *continuum*. Each new phase is built upon and connected to previous phases. The new phases are carefully planned *add-ons*. For example, one individual may wish to expand his or her social life. So instead of going to three meetings a week comprised on recovering alcoholics only, the individual goes to two of these meetings and begins to attend a church meeting comprised of church members.

By understanding that a life of sobriety is a continuum, the recovering alcoholic is not likely to drop the very things that have made for successful sobriety or take leaps to other activities that are really too challenging and not likely to be successful.

Focus on the Journey Not the Destination

One of the biggest traps or mistakes a recovering alcoholic can make is to expect to *arrive* at a high level of competence in attaining a healthy lifestyle. The problem is that the individual becomes consumed by the need to achieve a healthy lifestyle and then can become discouraged or disillusioned when setbacks occur, such as feeling quite bored or angry on occasions or making rushed decisions. The same issue could be put to a teacher, or any professional for that matter. For example, suppose we asked a teacher, "When do you become a perfect teacher?" The teacher would probably reply, "Never. But that is my goal. I see myself as a lifelong learner, always trying to improve my skills." Similarly, the quest for a healthy lifestyle can be likened to the quest for perfection. One never arrives at perfection but has a goal to be perfect and takes steps throughout a lifetime to keep improving.

The implication of this perspective is that recovering alcoholics should enjoy the experiences of an improved quality of life but should never rest on their laurels and say "I have arrived." Rather, the focus must be on the steps to systematically improve quality of life in an ongoing, lifelong manner.

Quality of Life is a Result Not a Strategy in Itself

A major goal for recovering alcoholics is to work toward a satisfying healthy lifestyle. A common mistake in this pursuit is to seek peace of mind, self-esteem, happiness, and other quality of life measures as things they can control directly. Consequently, when disturbances or interruptions to these pursuits occur (which we would call normal events to be expected), the individual feels failure and may become discouraged. The error lies in the individual's expectations that quality of life factors are things in their power to control. As the noted psychologist Viktor Frankl (1983) said, "But happiness cannot be pursued, it must ensue. One must have a reason to be happy. Once the reason is found, however, one becomes happy auto-matically" (p. 140). The approach recommended in this chapter is that recovering alcoholics can, and should, take charge of building skills that may lead to these quality of life results.

Emotional Sobriety

The concept of *emotional sobriety* and *dry drunk* are terms from the early Alcoholics Anonymous literature introduced by the founder Bill W (1988) to describe those individuals who have been very faithful to the AA program but who have not grown in important areas: "Since AA began, I've taken huge wallops in all these areas because of my failure to grow up, emotionally and spiritually" (*The Language of the Heart,* p. 236). Bill W appeals to the members of AA to address this critical area of focus in his thought-provoking letter as "The next frontier: Emotional sobriety," (236–238). He goes on to point out that a major factor limiting a person's growth in emotional maturity is connected to *dependence*: "Suddenly I realized what the matter was. My basic flaw had always been dependence—almost absolute depen-dence—on people or circumstances to supply me with prestige, security, and the like…" (p. 237).

The quest for emotional maturity, along with the concept of the dry drunk syndrome, speaks to the need to develop more skills following sobriety. It is clear that once a person achieves the gigantic accomplishment of becoming sober, the next question becomes "Can I accomplish more in my personal life beyond being sober?" The response is emphatically yes if sound procedural steps are taken to preserve sobriety and systematically target critical skill areas of personal growth.

Four Core Elements of Personal Growth

Growth in core areas of human nature is considered to be normal developmental occurrences through the passage of life and is typically used as an index of maturity in adults. Some individuals fail to grow in significant ways through, for example, on-going bad decisions affecting their lives in harmful ways or experiences with setbacks in life involving poor and destructive adjustments. Often these individuals systematically lose control of their lives leading to depression, melancholy, low self-esteem, and despair resulting in lifelong misery.

In a similar vein, alcoholics lose control of their lives, or, more accurately, alcohol begins to take control of their lives. This substantial loss of autonomy can also bring with it similar cognitive, social, and emotional problems and/or crises.

The recovering alcoholic can become free of alcohol through effective programs involving the support of others, be it fellowship in groups or personal contact with an individual. It is possible, in some cases, that the recovering alcoholic still manifests a high level of dependence. That is, there has been a shift from dependence on alcohol to dependence on the very structures that assisted the individual to become alcohol-free. This statement is not meant to be a criticism of the programs that assist individuals to become alcohol-free. It is indeed miraculous that such a turnaround can occur and occurs with high regularity. However, some recovering alcoholics may feel the need to take necessary measures to grow more in these areas that define their human nature. It is as if the recovering alcoholics have reached a "good level" and now seek a "better level" and not to let being sober alone limit their growth. This was poignantly recorded in an AA meeting involving Bill W: "Bill, haven't you often said right here in this meeting that sometimes the good is the enemy of the best?" (*Twelve Steps and Twelve Traditions*, p. 138).

The recovering alcoholic may well ask, "What are these needs you are talking about?" or "What is this healthy sobriety all about?" Section Three focuses on four major areas of our basic human makeup that are identified as the cornerstones of a healthy lifestyle: 1. Autonomous growth, 2. Cognitive growth, 3. Social growth, and 4. Emotional growth. These growth areas are now briefly described and will be developed more fully in Chapters 8, 9, 10, and 11 respectively.

> **Autonomous Growth** means all those factors that directly relate to the proper functioning and development of a person as an individual taking charge of his or her life while making decisions and solving problems. Other similar expressions include independence, self-reliance, personal responsibility, self-esteem, self-actualization, and problem-solving capacity.

> **Cognitive Growth** areas include all that is related to healthy and fruitful intellectual functioning or activities related to the mind such as reading, reflection, stimulating conversations, presentations, or written works, engaging movies, hobbies, and work or career activities.

> **Social Growth** refers to everything that involves healthy and productive interactions with other people which include conversations, working together,

making and keeping friends, relationships, friendly gatherings, outings, and joint activities.

Emotional Growth needs are those areas related essentially to feelings such as anger, joy, peace, fear, discomfort, anxiety, and optimism. Clearly, there is an array of feelings both positive and negative.

These four growth areas, while separated for discussion, really have no boundaries and are very interconnected. As one area expands, the other areas are also impacted in constructive ways. For example, if an individual experiences growth in managing emotions, the individual will also experience better clarity in managing decisions thereby growing in autonomy. This interconnectedness is depicted in Figure 7.1: Four Components for Personal Growth. Details for developing skills in these four areas are described in Chapters 8–11.

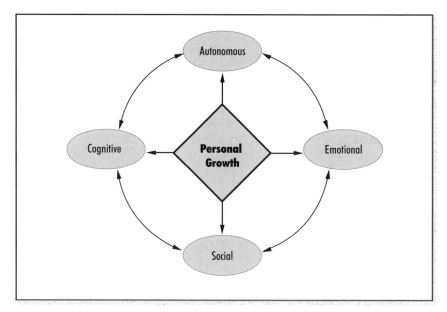

FIGURE 7.1: Four Components for Personal Growth

Pathway to Healthy Sobriety

Once sobriety has been attained, many recovering alcoholics face the challenge of how to enrich their lives—how to work toward *healthy sobriety*. To accomplish this additional goal, the pathway to sobriety needs also to include the dimension of personal growth for the pathway to lead to *healthy sobriety*. The following graph, Figure 7.2: Pathway to Healthy Sobriety, depicts the notion of competing pathways presented in Chapters 2–6, and, in addition, the representation of *growth* by the diamond inserted along the pathway to healthy sobriety. This diamond denotes the four key areas of *autonomous, cognitive, social,* and *emotional growth* briefly described above in Figure 7.1. Chapters 8–11 describe interventions for enabling personal growth in each of these four areas.

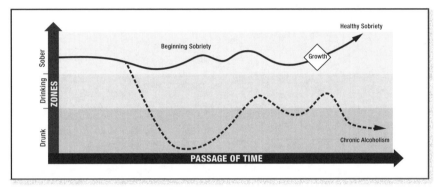

FIGURE 7.2: Pathway to Healthy Sobriety

Chapter Summary

There is no question that an extraordinary accomplishment has been achieved when an alcoholic quits drinking and is able to maintain sobriety. However, some recovering alcoholics then begin to ask the question, "Is there more to life than just being sober?" There appears to be a void in their lives and they begin to expect more enjoyment or fulfillment in their lives.

In this chapter, four crucial areas of human needs were pinpointed as necessary to fill this void or the hole within and enhance the quality of their life. These four areas of growth were identified as: *autonomous, cognitive, social,* and *emotional*.

While such growth can be seen as meritorious and satisfying, several important considerations were described to assist recovering alcoholics to understand what is involved in trying to lead a healthy life without jeopardizing their sobriety. It is particularly important for the recovering alcoholic to understand that this growth is really an extension of the alcohol-free lifestyle they have begun. It is not a replacement or something in opposition to the steps they have undertaken to achieve initial sobriety.

The primary goal is still to remain sober with added steps to systematically incorporate these four fundamental areas of growth: autonomous, social, cognitive, and emotional. Details for expanding and integrating each of these growth areas are presented in Chapters 8, 9, 10, and 11, respectively.

Skills for Autonomous Growth

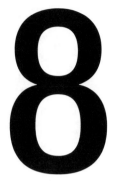

Happiness and freedom begin with a clear understanding of one principle: Some things are within our control, and some things are not. It is only after you have faced up to this fundamental rule and learned to distinguish between what you can and can't control that inner tranquility and outer effectiveness become possible.

— Epicetus

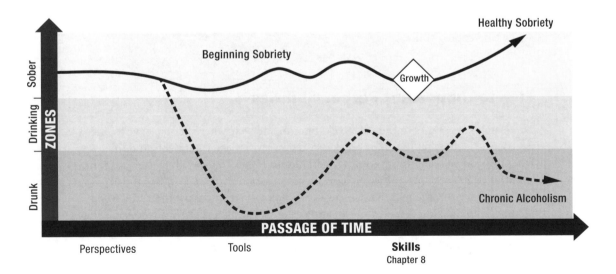

Alcoholism and autonomy are *polar opposites*. Alcoholics by definition have become dependent upon alcohol to the extent that alcohol begins to take control of them so that they gradually lose autonomy in most areas of their lives. Alcoholics in general need to free themselves from the yoke of alcoholism and develop a reasonable level of autonomy in their lives.

There are four components of personal growth leading to healthy sobriety—autonomous, cognitive, social, and emotional. The authors consider the first component, autonomous growth, an essential first step toward developing healthy sobriety, preventing relapses, and for setting the stage for growth in three other important areas of personal betterment (cognitive, social, and emotional, Chapters 9, 10, and 11, respectively).

One outcome of the process of achieving sobriety is that some alcoholics can become dependent on these structures and supports, not only to remain sober, but in other critical areas of their lives. Typically, many recovering alcoholics have lost the ability to make reasonable decisions, to know how to differentiate between what they want and what they need, and how to arrange things so there is some chance of getting what they need and want. Some recovering alcoholics yearn for more independence so that they can recover or rebuild autonomy in their lives without running the risk of losing their sobriety.

This chapter presents, in detail, the skills necessary for growth in autonomy and independence. The skill areas addressed are: 1. Plan for important responsibilities, 2. Solve problems effectively, 3. Kick the procrastination habit—*Do it now*, and 4. Develop coping skills.

Plan for Important Responsibilities

There are many points in the day, week, month, and year where people have to make decisions—from what to eat for breakfast to how to manage their debts and finances; from planning a menu to scheduling their day and week to meet all of their responsibilities. These responsibilities are considered to be a normal part of life and are addressed in a routine manner. However, alcoholics have often lost their way when it comes to managing responsibilities and certainly for planning ahead, considering options, and following through on their decisions. Alcoholics have simply learned to adapt in a world focused on drinking, getting drunk, recovering, and starting drinking again. Their planning and decision making became spur-of-the-moment actions and assumed secondary importance (with drinking being their primary focus). This means that the recovering alcoholic has to start from the beginning and learn how to make decisions, follow through on these decisions, and make plans. Essentially they have to learn how to take charge of their lives.

Develop Effective Routines

This is one of the most helpful ways of assisting a recovering alcoholic to make decisions and take charge of his or her life. Routines are those step-by-step procedures that a person follows for tasks or practices that occur on a regular basis such as getting ready for work, doing the laundry, cleaning the house, mapping out a schedule for the main activities for the week, and grocery shopping. The recovering alcoholic typically has very poor routines and planning in that they undertake the tasks in different ways each time, often leading to inefficiency and anxiety because the tasks do not get completed.

The following step-wise procedure is designed as a logical process for systematically teaching the skill of *establishing important routines* and becoming more autonomous by taking charge of things that need to be done. At first glance the steps may seem to be almost infantile and overkill. However, the basic premise is that a recovering alcoholic must learn how to take small steps toward autonomy in everything. These small, incremental steps are carefully designed to ensure that the individuals have the highest chance of being successful in taking charge of their day. The steps can be streamlined as the individual becomes more cognizant and practiced with the procedures.

A blank form for these steps is presented in the appendices section, Appendix E: Form 8.1, Procedural Steps for Developing Routines. An example is described in Illustration 8.1 which follows the explanations of the seven steps.

Step 1: Pinpoint a Difficult Responsibility and Get Started

This step in itself is a decision and marks in a significant manner that the recovering alcoholic wants to take charge of his or her life. It is understood that there is risk involved as the plan may or may not work satisfactorily and it is also understood that this method has been tried successfully with other individuals. The mere fact that the individual is making a decision to start indicates growth in autonomy right there.

In order to pinpoint a difficult responsibility the recovering alcoholics identify a time of the day, or responsibility, where they are usually struggling to do what is required. Ideally the initial target period occurs daily so that the individual can maintain focus and experience the effects of decisions on a frequent basis.

Step 2: Write Down How This Responsibility Is Usually Handled

For three consecutive days the individual writes down in a notebook each day everything that happens during this period—the routine that is followed, problems that may arise, any feelings that may emerge, decisions that are made, or changes that occur from one period to the next.

Step 3. Write Down a Specific Routine for This Period

The individual maps out in a step-by-step manner the routine that will be followed so that all the necessary responsibilities are met.

Step 4: Implement the Routine for Three Consecutive Days

The planned routine is now implemented for three consecutive days. The individual takes note at the earliest opportunity of whether or not each step in the routine is followed.

Step 5: Adapt the Routine as Necessary

The individual may find some steps are not efficient or are too difficult. In these cases the steps need to be changed to something that is more workable.

Step 6: Evaluate the Effectiveness of the Routine

After the plan has been implemented for at least a week, including minor changes, the individual evaluates the effectiveness of the plan. The basic question comes down to "Is the responsibility getting done in a reasonable way now?" If the answer is *yes* then the individual maintains the plan. If the answer is *no* then the routine needs to be adjusted by making changes in the steps of the routine.

Step 7: Plan for Other Areas of Responsibilities

Once the individual has experienced success with the first routine it is a much smaller step now to target other areas of responsibilities by following the same steps (Steps 1–8). As time progresses, individuals will more than likely experience growth in awareness of what planning they need to develop to meet their responsibilities during their day and, most importantly, will begin to experience that they can indeed take charge of these targeted areas. Moreover, the individuals will then be able to approach any period during the day and develop a plan to increase their autonomy in this period. A blank form for Illusration 8.1 is presented in Appendix E: Form 8.1, Procedural Steps for Developing Routines.

Background: Sara is a 37-year-old teacher assistant in a Christian Pre-School Center. She is separated from her husband and has no children. Her support system includes a church-based recovery group which meets twice a week for study using the Recovery Bible and her mother keeps in close contact. She was a heavy drinker for many years and became an alcoholic over the past 5 years. Her husband left her because of her drinking issues. Through her friends in the church she has been able to quit drinking and maintain a job. She is looking at her lifestyle more closely now that she has been sober for just over 18 months.

ILLUSTRATION 8.1: Procedural Steps for Developing Routines

Step 1: Pinpoint a difficult responsibility and get started.
I would like to feel that I can take charge of my life. My friends seem to be doing this. I want that. I think the start of a workday would be good place to start. I am alone in the mornings and won't have outside interruptions. I have an awful time getting going and often get to work a little late and in a mad rush—not a good way to start the work day especially for the children.

Step 2: Write down how this responsibility is usually handled.
The alarm goes off. I feel so tired that I hit the snooze button several times. I don't go back to sleep; I just lie there with my mind wandering all over. Then I do get out of bed and sit on the bed wondering what I will do next. I go to the bathroom, think I will make the coffee then I decide to get the paper. I start to read the paper then think I need some coffee but there are no clean cups. I decide to get ready for work, but I don't know what to wear so I start to make the bed. The sheets need laundering, so I take a shower at that point and get dressed and grab some coffee on the way to work. When I finally get to work I am just glad to be out of the house, but when I get home I run into the usual mess in the bedroom and kitchen. And so it goes.

ILLUSTRATION 8.1 *Continued*

Step 3: Write down a specific routine for this period.

- *Set my clothes out the night before*
- *Get up when the alarm goes off and go straight to the kitchen and make coffee*
- *Get the paper*
- *Prepare breakfast*
- *Eat breakfast, read the paper, and drink coffee*
- *Clean up after breakfast—wash dishes and put everything away*
- *Shower*
- *Dress*
- *Make the bed and pick up in bedroom*
- *Close the house and head to work*

Step 4: Adapt the routine as necessary.

I made one change. I found that when I got the paper I started reading it immediately and didn't get to preparing breakfast and started up on my old ways of jumping around. So I got the paper after I had breakfast ready (changed step 3 in the routine to step 5). This worked great.

Step 5: Implement the routine for three consecutive days.

I followed the new routine for three days and wrote down how I did. It was straight forward really and by the third day I felt I was on auto.

Step 6: Evaluate the effectiveness of the routine.

It became very clear that the new routine worked well because I was on time for work each day, felt more relaxed, engaged the children immediately, and I got to come home to a clean kitchen and bedroom which helps me to relax at home. It was obvious to me that I was on a roll and didn't have to think too much about what to do next. It was like I was on automatic.

Step 7: Plan for other areas of responsibilities.

I developed a routine for dinner and made a schedule for important things that had to be done for the week and posted it in the kitchen.

Solve Problems Effectively

A second area concerning autonomous growth is the ability to solve problems. Alcoholics are often characterized by an inability to face problems. Drinking more alcohol has been the adopted strategy when problems arise, which of course compounds problems rather than solves them. Once recovering alcoholics become more proficient in solving problems, they experience growth in autonomy by taking charge of their lives.

Again, a key assumption is that problem solving is a skill that can be learned and that the skill can be broken down into discrete teachable steps. Variations of the following steps for teaching problem solving can be found in the literature (Colvin, 2009; Ellis 2001; Gorski, 1989; Monti, Abrams, Kadden, & Cooney, 1989).

In this model an eight-step procedure is used to teach problem-solving skills.

Step 1: Recognize the Problem

This initial step involves the individual coming to terms with the fact there is indeed a problem. On the surface this may seem to be an obvious, if not inconsequential, step. Wrong. Alcoholics have learned to live with problems and have become inured to them through long periods of denial. It would be like a person living in a fog and getting used to that range of visibility. They lose sight of what it would be like to live outside of this fog and see with clarity.

Problems are typically recognized through feedback of one sort or another that can be manifested and categorized the following ways:

- **Physical ailments** such as: stomach aches, migraines, fatigue, and lack of sleep

- **Emotional factors** involving regular negative feelings such as despair, depression, anxiety, fear, and loneliness

- **Concerns from others** such as ongoing comments from family members, friends, and other recovering alcoholics

- **Loss of skills and interests,** noticing that there are many things that they are not able to do now that used to be part of their lifestyle

- **Repercussions** may have occurred from drinking days that have forced the person into an unsatisfying job or unemployment, struggling relationships, and financial hardship.

In starting out, the individual may identify *several problems* and wonder where to start or perhaps become overcome and discouraged with how much has to be addressed. In these cases the individual needs to select *one problem only* to get started. It might be best to select a problem that occurs daily or is foremost on their mind. Other problems can be addressed at a later stage.

Step 2: Clarify the Problem

In this step the individual clearly pinpoints what is going on in concrete and specific ways. Details are noted addressing key questions such as who, what, when, where, and why. Other people, family, friends, support personnel such as sponsors, can also help with identifying the specifics of the nature of the problem. The individual needs to be able to say at the end of this step something like "Yes I am having a problem getting along with people at work" or "I don't see eye to eye with my wife and we are having lots of arguments" or "I get terribly restless and worried after dinner in the evening."

Step 3: Identify Explanations for the Problem

This step involves taking a good look at possible reasons for the particular problem. Once these reasons have been indentified, it becomes easier to select strategies for solving the problem. For example, an individual may have trouble getting along with a workmate or supervisor because of a long history of conflict. The solution might be to sit down and identify this conflict as a cause of problems and reach some agreement about "burying the hatchet" and taking a fresh start. This step helps the individual to connect the problem-solving strategy to the causes of the problem.

Step 4: List Intervention Options

At this juncture, many recovering alcoholics will want to rush in and fix the problem. They may impulsively take the first solution available, implement it, and it may not be successful. It is better to take a more measured approach and list a number of options. The recommended approach is to simply brainstorm and write down all the possible solutions to this problem that could be used.

Step 5: Select the Most Favorable Option

Now the individual is in a position to select a strategy to try to solve the specific problem. Again caution must be used. It is critical for the individual to weigh the various options and determine which one is most likely to be successful. Some considerations that should be addressed are:

- Is the strategy affordable?

- Do I have time to do it?

- Is it something that can be done fairly soon versus down the road?

- Is it something I can do myself or will I need help? (And, if help is needed, is someone lined up to provide the help?)

- Is it something I can readily do or will I have to learn more skills?

The individual then selects a strategy that is a best fit to these kinds of questions.

Step 6: Implement Intervention

Now it is time for action, this is where "the rubber hits the road." Quite often a recovering alcoholic will show great participation and enthusiasm for Steps 1–5 but may balk at implementing the plan, Step 6. The recovering alcoholic (and support person if involved) must realize that this step is both challenging and daunting. It is probably a pathway that the individual has not taken for quite some time. He or she can expect some fear and worry about success. In many cases the individual will need strong encouragement to undertake this step. Helpful comments at this point might be "You've come this far. Let's do it" or "You can do it" or "Look, give it a try.

If it works, great. If not, we will try something else. There are plenty of things we can do."

Step 7: Evaluate Effectiveness

Once the problem-solving strategy has been implemented—for 2 to 3 weeks at least, it is very important to evaluate the procedure. The key questions are:

- Is it working or not?

- Have there been any changes in the situation?

- Has the situation worsened, remained the same, or improved?

Step 8: Decide to Maintain, Modify, or Change Intervention

Once the strategy has been evaluated in terms of its effectiveness, decisions need to be made on whether to maintain the strategy, modify the plan, or develop a new plan.

Maintain the strategy. It may be that some gains are being made and that it would be worth continuing with the plan. Also, the individual may not have followed through with the plan in a consistent manner and time is needed to give the strategy a reasonable chance of being effective.

Modify the plan. Some slight changes to the plan may be needed. Perhaps the plan needs to involve less time (or more time), to be implemented more often, or to have some other pieces added to the plan.

Develop a new plan. It is concluded that the plan did not work and that another plan is needed. In this case the individual (and support person as appropriate) would return to Steps 3–7. It is very important that when a plan is dropped, the individual does not feel he or she has failed. Rather the plan was not effective and a new one is needed. That is *the plan has failed, not the individual.*

A blank form this procedure is presented in the appendices section, Appendix F: Form 8.2, Procedural Steps for Solving Problems Effectively, and an example of the procedures is described in Illustration 8.2.

Background: Jon, a 46-year-old single man, after 27 years of short periods of sobriety followed by longer and longer periods of active drinking, elected to go to a state-sponsored treatment center and then join AA. He has been very active in AA while living in a halfway house. He has found a job working part-time as a mover for a furniture store. Two months ago he moved into a studio from the halfway house. With vouchers from the Salvation Army he has been able to furnish the quad. He has food stamps at this time but hopes soon to be self-supporting. He is doing well at work but is becoming increasingly restless with his living situation.

ILLUSTRATION 8.2: Procedural Steps for Solving Problems Effectively

Step 1: Recognize the problem.
I have been feeling real nervous and restless in the last month. Not sure what is going on. I am happy with my place, but I don't feel settled. I have been looking forward to my own place, but it just isn't right. I don't feel that it's my home. I spend most of my time somewhere else. My money runs out very quickly too.

Step 2: Clarify the problem.
It became clear to me that the root problem was that I cannot cook. So I eat out a lot which ends up being a big expense (no wonder I run out of money).I need to learn how to cook more than one meal..

Step 3: Identify explanations for the problem.
I never learned to cook as I have led a traveling existence. I have been on the streets for years and the only real meals I got were either at the mission or in jail. In the half-way house when it was my turn to cook, I either made spaghetti or chili and I sure am tired of just this. Basically with my lifestyle I have never learned to cook.

Step 4: List intervention options.
1) I could go to cooking school.
2) I could ask the county extension office for material on cooking.
3) I could get a cookbook and learn that way.
4) I could just go on the way I am and add a new meal from time to time.
5) I could ask some of the single guys at AA how they cook for themselves.

Step 5: Select the most favorable option.
I knew I had very limited cash so I chose calling the county extension office and seems like they have pamphlets on just about anything. They had a prepared bundle on basic nutrition, setting up a kitchen, grocery shopping, and simple recipes for some basic meals. About two weeks' worth. Also I thought I could get started this way and ask questions of my buddies at AA as needed.

ILLUSTRATION 8.2 *Continued*

Step 6: Implement intervention.

I got the information from the county but just the titles seemed daunting. There was so much to do. But I kept challenging my negative mind. I would find a way. So I compromised and just looked at the pamphlet on setting up a kitchen and checked to see how I was managing my kitchen. There were one or two things missing I got those and went on. Again, the grocery shopping seemed like too much, but I had a friend from AA help me simplify the list. After a while that was okay and the cooking was less difficult than I thought. I learned the trick is knowing what to cook. I prepared 5 meals at home for the week (hamburgers, sausages, pasta dishes, and fish dinners). I had sandwich fixings for lunch and cereal, toast, and coffee for breakfast.

Step 7: Evaluate effectiveness.

Not even a month went by before I knew that I can actually cook a decent meal, and when I go to the grocery store I know what I am about. It is a good feeling to know what you are doing. Besides my food stamps go farther if I follow the suggestions in the book. In the last month I have even dropped some weight. I eat better, feel better, and it is funny but I feel like I am the boss in the kitchen and I am enjoying my studio now and don't feel the need to get out like I did. I even had my AA buddy over for dinner—my first guest for dinner since I quit drinking.

Step 8: Decide to maintain, modify, or change intervention.

This is working. I am going to maintain it. The only modification that I implemented during the month was in planning the menu. I just could not afford either time-wise or money-wise to have a different meal each day. So I now plan 4 meals a week with left-overs for 3 days. This will save time and money. I really feel that the cooking has made me more independent and much more settled at home.

Kick the Procrastination Habit—Do It Now

It is one thing for recovering alcoholics to come to terms with what decisions they should make during the course of a day and to develop problem-solving skills. However, each of these skills requires that the individuals make these decisions *in a timely manner*. Recovering alcoholics are often prone to delaying decisions or avoiding them outright. This failure to make decisions in a timely manner is called *procrastination*.

The purpose of this section is to provide information to assist recovering alcoholics in developing skills for making decisions on time and in avoiding the destructive habit of procrastination in general. The topics addressed are: 1. Description and causes of procrastination, and 2. General guidelines and specific strategies for overcoming procrastination and building self-regulation.

Description and Causes of Procrastination

Procrastination is the practice of needlessly putting off things that need to be done immediately. Granted, it is part of human nature to delay responding to certain things that are aversive to us, such as returning a call to someone who is angry at us or putting off laundry because there is a good movie on TV. However, we are using procrastination in the sense of a *habit* where an individual predictably avoids decisions and actions that should not be delayed. For some people, particularly recovering alcoholics, procrastination has become a way of life. They operate in a state of inertia when decisions have to be made and simply freeze for a host of reasons. Consequently, decisions do not get made or get made way too late. These individuals live in a state of *avoidance* and spend a considerable amount of time and energy trying to mop up after important decisions have not been made. By contrast, the desirable habit, in opposition to procrastination, is self-regulation where things are done in a *timely* and *planned* manner. In general, procrastination has quite harmful, long-term effects on an individual's quality of life: careers are impacted, social relationships are diminished, and the individuals' self-esteem and self-worth are significantly reduced.

There are many serious, harmful, and deleterious effects resulting from procrastination. These effects reach into many corners of an individual's life when procrastination becomes habitual behavior. Their negative effects include: problems with relationships, health issues, missed opportunities, and financial losses (Steel, 2007).

> **Weakens Relationships.** Once individuals assume the habit of not getting things done, it is not long before family members, friends, and workmates lose respect for them and end up excluding them from important events and processes. Procrastinators assume a role of being irresponsible and untrustworthy, causing others to work around them or without them. They become excluded.

> **Health Issues.** Taking care of one's health requires fidelity to a number of decisions and actions. For example, the individual needs to eat appropriately which implies planning menus and shopping accordingly. These activities typically do not occur with the habitual procrastinator. Similarly, an individual can experience mental health issues when so much time, energy, and emotion is spent on trying to clean things up later because the things were not done or were delayed. This heightened stress following procrastination

can also trigger relapses where the individual resumes drinking alcohol to get relief from the stress. A delay in seeking medical advice could mean the difference between life and death.

Missed Opportunities The individual who is slow to respond to opportunities will clearly be left behind by those who respond on time. Individuals who do not get reports in on time, are late for meetings, and consistently delay making decisions with others waiting on those

> **"Procrastination is the grave of opportunity"**
> (author unknown)

decisions will not last long in the workforce (at least in that position). *Procrastinator* is a label that will hold a person back in the workforce and will certainly deny individuals opportunities in other areas of life as well.

Financial Losses. Procrastination with its bedfellow disorganization can lead to substantial financial losses. For example, people pay more in taxes because of procrastination with filing returns; individuals pay late fees because bills are not paid on time or items such as movies or books are not returned on time; services are discontinued because of habitual late payments. Individuals with poor management skills often are not covered for emergencies and do not have retirement plans.

Causes of Procrastination

The habit of procrastination can be established for any number of reasons. While the root causes of procrastination may vary from individual to individual, it is helpful to consider the common factors which should be addressed when replacing this habit with self-regulation skills required for getting things done on time. The common root causes include already established bad habits from alcoholism, expectation of immediate gratification, faulty thinking, destructive emotions, and disorganization.

Carryover from Alcoholism. When individuals are controlled by alcoholism, one of the significant damaging outcomes is the lost capacity to make decisions and take charge of their lives. Typically, alcoholics are either preoccupied or occupied with drinking day and night. This addiction makes it very difficult, if not impossible, for individuals to make decisions to get things that need to be done, done on time (or even done at all). The alcoholic loses all sense of prioritizing responsibilities with the result that ongoing important decisions are not made or made far too late. Consequently, when individuals become sober they can expect to experience difficulty when it comes to organizing their lives proactively and in making decisions in a timely manner. In effect, they have developed a bad habit of procrastination which obviously needs to be addressed for healthy sobriety to occur.

Immediate Gratification. Individuals establish and maintain various bad habits that give them immediate reinforcement, gratification, or relief from their actions. With procrastination, the individuals are reinforced by either obtaining relief, albeit short term, from not having to do something they do not wish to do, or gratification from doing something else that is more pleasurable at the time, such as watching a movie when they should be doing their grocery shopping. We take the position that through this *avoidance-reinforcement* paradigm, procrastination is a learned behavior and that its opposite partner, doing things in a timely manner, can also be learned.

Faulty Thinking. The individual may overestimate or underestimate the amount of time needed to perform a task. Quite often recovering alcoholis think they need to be in the right mood to do something and have to wait for that mood to arrive. They may feel they are not presently equipped to complete the task and need to wait for more information or more resources to be available. Similarly, they may be perfectionists and need to have endless details in place before beginning or will not begin until they are assured that everything will proceed perfectly.

Destructive Emotions. Emotions play an important role in establishing and maintaining the habit of procrastination. Individuals who are driven by *fear*, especially, become quite creative in avoiding decisions and waiting until it is too late to make the decisions. Fear of failure, fear of what others think, feelings of inadequacy and discouragement can cause an individual to retreat when decision-making time comes. Soon the alcoholic and recovering alcoholic become embroiled with procrastination so that tasks and responsibilities build up. This situation can then lead to the all-consuming emotion of *depression*. Depression, if not effectively addressed, can bury the individual in procrastination.

Disorganization. The alcoholic and organization are terms not usually associated (unless we are talking about planning for access to alcohol). During the period when individuals became consumed with alcohol, they usually lose their organizational skills simply because most of their life events and needs became unimportant. Consequently, when an individual becomes sober, these events and needs become more important, but the needed skills are absent. The individual has learned to live in a dysfunctional and disorganized manner. It is almost impossible to determine which decisions need to be made and when to make them when the individual's life is chaotic and disorganized. Clearly, a major step toward dealing with procrastination for recovering alcoholics is to restore some order and organization to their lives.

General Guidelines and Specific Strategies for Overcoming Procrastination and Building Self-Regulation

The approach here for overcoming procrastination is to assume that the recovering alcoholic has learned a bad habit and that through systematic steps new habits can be learned (or re-learned as the case may be) to make decisions in a timely manner. The primary focus for overcoming procrastination is to assist recovering alcoholics with managing their affairs in a timely manner, basically to manage their to-do lists. Some of the specific strategies for learning these new skills may work for some and not for others. The basic message to recovering alcoholics is that they will surely find something that works for them if they keep working with the guidelines and trying different strategies to find what works best for them. Persistence is the key.

The following information is presented for overcoming the habit of procrastination and developing the habit of self-regulation: 1. General guidelines to overcoming procrastination habits, and 2. Specific steps for managing to-do lists.

General Guidelines to Overcoming Procrastination Habits

Exercise Firm Resolve. As with any significant personal change, the beginning step must be a firm resolve to do what it takes to succeed. Recovering alcoholics will surely remember the time when they made a commitment to quit drinking. This step was not taken lightly and was made with a certain amount of trepidation. However, the individual was well aware that the decision to quit drinking had to be made and made with firm resolve. Moreover, recovering alcoholics can now take comfort in that they have been successful with the formidable challenge to change from being an alcoholic to becoming a *recovering* alcoholic. They have quit alcohol. Now they must turn their energy and resolve to beat the bad habit of procrastination and develop self-regulation skills and practices.

Get Started and Stay with It. This is where the rubber hits the road. That is, when the recovering alcoholic has to do what is on the list at the time specified in the schedule. A number of tips are available to help a person get started with a task and to stay with it until the task is completed.

Anticipate Self-Distractions. Individuals need to be ready for the little procrastination games they are likely to play. For example, it is on the schedule to do the laundry and Thomas thinks "Oh I had better make a phone call or I may miss him" or "I had better check my email as I am expecting an important message." It is helpful to use some self-talk in these situations such as "There I go trying to put off the laundry. I can do the laundry. I will do the laundry." The distractions, in this case making the phone call or checking email, can then be used as a reward for when the laundry task is completed.

Start with Easy Tasks. Sometimes it is hard for an individual to take on a difficult task or a task that takes considerable time. In these cases it can be useful to begin with an easy task. In this way the individual is producing, following through with what's on the schedule, and successfully completing the task. The more difficult task is scheduled to follow completion of this easier task. The easy task helps the individual gain some momentum and thereby overcomes the reluctance to get started with the more difficult task. For example, doing the laundry is a difficult task because it takes so long. So Thomas felt the urge to make a phone call when he was about to start the laundry. He decided to take out the garbage instead, a short and easy task, which was followed by getting underway with the laundry. The easy task of taking out the garbage helped to displace the need for the phone call and made it easier for him to then get underway with the laundry.

Use Avoidance or Preferred Activities as Rewards. One way of addressing distractions that arise when a task is to be managed is to use them as rewards for finishing the task. The distraction is typically a preferred activity such as watching some TV, making a phone call, or getting online. So rather than yielding to the distraction of completing the task (procrastination), the individual completes the task and then (as a reward) engages in the activity that posed as a distraction. For example, when Thomas was due to do the laundry, he thought he should make a phone call. However, he decided to complete the laundry job and then make the phone call. In this way making the phone call not only serves as a reward for finishing the laundry, he will be much more relaxed and satisfied when making the call because he was successful in completing the laundry task.

Focus on the Details of the Task Rather Than Your Thoughts. Individuals who are prone to procrastination often have their minds full of all sorts of thoughts before they begin a task. These thoughts can cause the individual to stop the task, reconsider, or choke. Regardless, the thoughts can easily control the actions of the individual. One strategy for dealing with the power of thoughts is to directly focus on the details of the task at hand. Essentially, one cannot think of two things at once, so by concentrating on some aspect of the task, the mind is then occupied and the distracting thoughts are pre-empted or displaced. For example, when Thomas was about to start doing the laundry, he began to think of all the phone calls he needed to make and what would happen if he didn't make them. He also thought of emails he might be getting and what he would do if he did not get certain ones. In effect, these thoughts were taking over. His first step in doing the laundry was to sort his clothes. He began to look more closely at his shirts as he sorted them thinking one shirt is holding up well and maybe another shirt could be given to Goodwill as it is too big for him. The focus and thoughts on laundry details helped him to remove the distracting thoughts about phone calls and emails. He was then able to stay with the laundry task.

Break Tasks Down into Smaller Tasks. One reason recovering alcoholics procrastinate is that a task is just too overwhelming. They just cannot get started because they are not sure where to start or where to go next. One way of addressing this problem is to break a big task down into a number of smaller tasks. For example, if the house is a mess and needs cleaning, the individual could plan to clean one room at a time. Or if a particular room is a mess, the tasks could be broken down into areas, such as tidy up the countertops first, then the bed, then the floor, and so on. Breaking a big task into smaller tasks provides the individual with a sharper focus, helps the individual to experience closure once each small step is completed, and helps to provide a roadmap for the whole task.

Managing Breaks. On the surface it is reasonable for an individual to take a break when longer tasks are involved. However, taking a break can be a trap. Individuals can begin to use breaks as an escape strategy when difficulties arise with the task they need to complete, resulting in the job not getting done. Given a break is needed, it is best to plan the break ahead of time. For example, to take a break after items on the bed and floor are picked up and put away. In addition, limits should be set on how long the break should be. Ideally, a short break is planned so that it is not too difficult to return to completing the rest of the task on the schedule. For example, Julie decides to take a break and work on the crossword for 10 minutes after she has picked up and put away the surface areas in her bedroom.

Specific Strategies for Managing the To-Do List

Alcoholics typically lose a sense of priorities and for managing their affairs in a timely manner so that when they quit alcohol, they have to learn or re-learn these skills. In this section six steps are described for teaching recovering alcoholics to take charge of their affairs by managing their to-do lists. A blank planning form for these steps is presented in the appendices section, Appendix G: Form 8.3, Planning Guide for Managing To-Do Lists. An example of a plan using this form is described in Illustration 8.3 following a description of the steps.

Step 1: List the To-Do Tasks

This list is comprised of all the things that an individual needs to take care of for normal, healthy living, such as doing the laundry, getting a haircut, and paying bills. Step 1 involves having the recovering alcoholic simply make a list of what needs to be done. At this stage there is no need to worry about which ones should be on the list or which ones should be done first. The step is simply to list the tasks. Also, it is important that the items on the list are concrete tasks rather than generalities. For example, it is better to put down *take a walk or ride the bike* rather than do some *exercise*. Generalities can often lead to procrastination whereas if the item on the list is concrete, then the individual does not have to think that much around what needs to be done and all the options available.

Step 2: Prioritize the List

Clearly some items are more important than others. For example, it is probably more important to do the grocery shopping if one is out of food compared to going to the library to get some more books. A simple strategy for prioritizing the to-do list is to rank each item on a scale of 1 through 3 where 1 means somewhat important, 2 means important and 3 means very important. Once the list is completed the individual rates each item 1 through 3.

Step 3: Develop a Schedule

Once the to-do list has been developed and prioritized the next step is to determine when these tasks will be undertaken. The recovering alcoholic determines roughly how long a task might take and then considers when the tasks could be done. Some tasks can be quite challenging because they take a considerable amount of time while others may be easier because they only take a little time. Tasks need also to be ranked, 1 through 3, according to the estimated time for completion where 1 means a short task, 2 means a medium task, and 3 means a long task. In Appendix G: Form 8.3, Guidelines for Managing To-Do Lists, the recovering alcoholic or support person is asked to underline the appropriate rating of the length for each task (1 through 3) in the schedule column and then writes in a date and a time based on the rating of the task length. Sometimes it is helpful to intersperse some of the short tasks with the long tasks to avoid overwhelming the recovering alcoholic.

The importance of this step cannot be overstated. The mere fact that the recovering alcoholic, who is struggling with procrastination, writes down when a task will be undertaken is a step in the right direction. Obviously, writing it down does not ensure that it gets done, but the step provides a jolt or reminder for the alcoholic and becomes part of the *resolve* to do what needs to be done.

Step 4: Check for Completion

One of the surest ways of knowing whether or not an individual is beginning to overcome procrastination is to determine whether a designated task has been completed or not. In some cases, an individual's struggle with procrastination is mostly centered on getting started. However, procrastination also applies to finishing a task. Individuals may get started and then find creative ways of stopping before the task is completed. This step is designed to remind the individual that a task needs not only to be started in a timely manner but also finished in a timely manner. To determine the status of a task completed or not we recommend a *Yes* or *No* response. A *Yes* response means that the task is entirely finished. Even if the individual has completed 90% of the task, the recorded response would be *No*. It is not recorded as a *Yes* until it is fully completed.

Step 5: Reschedule as Needed

In the event that a task is not finished in the scheduled time, this task should be rescheduled at the next available opportunity. Reasons why the task was not completed should be recorded in the next column, Step 6, Review. Some reasons could be that the individual did not allow sufficient time for the task; there were unplanned interruptions, for example, a friend dropping by; the individual may have entertained multiple distractions and puttered along with the task; or there may have been unforeseen problems that needed to be addressed. The key is to reschedule the task at the next reasonable opportunity.

Step 6: Review

This step can be very helpful to recovering alcoholics as they begin the process for developing the skills of self-regulation. During their days of alcoholism, it is highly likely that they learned many bad habits when it came to managing their affairs. The kinds of items that are recorded in this step are meant to be helpful for future occasions as the individual is developing new habits. Entries might include: adjustments to the tasks; details of tasks broken down into smaller steps; what made getting started hard; what distractions occur; how breaks were taken; or any aspect in conflict with following the suggested guidelines. This step also helps to keep the individual accountable. Finally, the step is very similar to the recommendations made earlier in this book for the recovering alcoholic to keep a running journal.

A blank form for these guidelines is presented in the Appendix G: Form 8.3, Guidelines for Managing To-Do Lists, and an example is described in Illustration 8.3.

Background: Monique has been incarcerated for 36 months from charges stemming from an automobile accident in which her son was seriously injured. Monique was drinking at the time of the accident. She began in college and continued until the accident. She had never lost a job, but her husband had complained for years about her drinking and that the house was a mess and she was always disorganized. While she was in prison, her husband divorced her, taking their son to live in another state. She quit drinking and began attending meetings while she was incarcerated. She met another inmate who had recovered using the Rational Recovery Program. She soon became an enthusiastic practitioner of Rational Emotive Therapy. When released she went back to school to learn computer programming. In meeting with her parole officer, she realized how disorganized she was and the need to do something about it. Her PO said she uses a planning list or a to-do list to get everything done. Monique decided to develop a to-do list.

ILLUSTRATION 8.3: Planning Guide for Managing To-Do Lists

Step 1 To-Do List List tasks to be done	Step 2 Priority (Underline) 1: Somewhat Important 2: Important 3: Very Important	Step 3 Scheduled for (Underline) 1: Short Task 2: Medium task 3: Long task	Step 4 Completed (Underline) Yes or No	Step 5 Rescheduled for	Step 6 Review Note any explanations, successes, decisions, or insights
Haircut	<u>1</u> 2 3	1 <u>2</u> 3 Date: *Thurs. 11/12* Time: *5 pm*	<u>Yes</u> No	Date: Time:	*Scheduled the haircut for straight after class which had become a void time since I quit drinking.*
Laundry	1 <u>2</u> 3	1 <u>2</u> 3 Date: *Weekly* Time: *Sat. am*	Yes <u>No</u>	Date: *Wed. evening* Time: *6 pm*	*Laundromat was packed so switched to Wednesday evening during dinner time.*
Tidy house	1 <u>2</u> 3	1 2 <u>3</u> Date: *Daily* Time: *Before dinner*	<u>Yes</u> No	Date: Time:	
Grocery shop-ping	1 2 <u>3</u>	1 2 <u>3</u> Date: *Weekly* Time: *Sat. am*	Yes <u>No</u>	Date: *Sun.* Time: *am*	*Friend was visiting Sat. am so rescheduled for first thing Sun. am.*
Write letter to son	1 2 <u>3</u>	1 2 <u>3</u> Date: *Weekly* Time: *Tues. eve*	Yes <u>No</u>	Date: *Wed.* Time: *After dinner*	*Found it too hard to write—fear he didn't like me. Words don't come easy. Decided to send a post card to at least say hello—that worked for me. I then scheduled to send a card next week. I think I can do that now– a card with a short note.*

Develop Coping Skills

The earlier sections of this chapter for addressing autonomous growth focused on those areas that an individual can directly control: take charge where necessary, solve problems effectively, and do it now and don't procrastinate. Each of these areas has one key assumption and that is the individual can, through his or her efforts, *change the situation*. However, there are many situations in people's lives, including the lives of recovering alcoholics, where individuals experience deep concern and are not able to change the situation such as: the troublesome behavior of a relative; the ongoing noise and inconsideration of neighbors; a job that is boring and frustrating; health issues and limitations that are permanent; and personal tragedies. In some cases these situations were the reasons or the kinds of reasons the individual may have turned to alcohol in the first place. The question becomes "How can an individual learn to manage the events so that he or she can function at a reasonable level without becoming too upset and, worse still, turning to alcohol for relief?"

As with the rest of Section Three the approach is to assume that individuals need to learn skills for dealing with these situations that they cannot directly control or manipulate. These are called *coping skills*. The topics addressed in this section are: 1. Description of coping skills, 2. Assessing the situation, 3. Coping skill strategies, and 4. Checklist and action plan for coping skills.

Description of Coping Skills

Coping skills are those strategies that enable individuals to overcome or offset the negative effects of adverse conditions without removing or changing the underlying factors. Certain situations become very difficult for individuals. This can cause considerable stress. Through effective coping skills, individuals learn how to minimize the stress and anxiety that these situations may cause with the expectation that the situation itself will not change. For example, an individual may have an obnoxious workmate who causes considerable stress (the workmate happens to be the boss's son). The individual learns ways to minimize contact with this person and limits interactions solely to specific work tasks. The focus is totally on the work and not on any personal interactions between them. Otherwise, the individual gives this workmate a wide berth. Negative examples of coping skills, would be to engage in confrontations with this person, talk negatively to other workmates, seek ways to make this person pay, or quit an otherwise satisfactory and much needed job. The result of such negative approaches is usually counterproductive and brings about more stress for the individual as Pavrajika Vrajaprana (1999) aptly noted:

> Our thoughts and actions aren't so much arrows as boomerangs— eventually they find their way back home. (p. 10)

Note: It is imperative for recovering alcoholics to learn coping skills for these uncontrollable and unchanging situations not only to manage their stress level but also to avoid the possibility of a relapse. Individuals who have used alcohol in the past as a coping strategy are highly likely to return to drinking (Morgenstern & Longabaugh, 2000), which will be discussed more fully in Chapter 12: Addressing Relapses.

Assessing the Situation

As with any intervention, assessments need to be made to determine which interventions should be used and which ones may not be appropriate. The key information needed is whether the situation is something that can be controlled or changed. If the assessment indicates that the situation can be changed, then *problem-solving strategies* described earlier in this chapter should be used. Or, if the assessment shows that the situation is uncontrollable or unchangeable, then *coping strategies* need to be used. Typically, the individual would make such a judgment by examining the situation or discussing the matter with a support person (friend, relative, counselor, or sponsor).

After reaching the assessment that the situation is uncontrollable and unchangeable a second determination needs to be made whether or not the situation can be left. If it is possible and desirable to withdraw from the situation, the individual should do so as soon as practical. However, if the individual cannot withdraw from the situation and is stuck with it, then coping skills need to be developed and implemented.

Coping Skill Strategies

Once it has been determined that the problem situation is one that is uncontrollable or unchangeable, the recovering alcoholic needs to use coping skills. These skills provide the individuals with ways of strengthening themselves so that they can withstand the impact of the problem situation. Given the individuals are "stuck with" the problem situation, the following practices are designed to enable them to lead reasonably healthy lifestyles.

Accept the Situation

First and foremost, given withdrawal is not an option, the recovering alcoholic must accept that the situation *cannot be changed* and that he or she has to live with it. Alcoholics Anonymous has institutionalized this concept with the adoption of the *Serenity Prayer:*

> ...[T]he serenity to accept the things I cannot change, courage to change the things I can, and wisdom to know the difference.

Related to the notion of accepting the situation is the concept of letting go. Even though the situation bothers them, they need to show detachment and avoid perseverating on the situation since there is nothing they can do about it. Simply let it go.

Manage the Moment

There are usually two windows for coping with problem situations. The first is when the problem is truly present, for example when a person is working in a hostile environment. The second is outside of the situation, such as the times before or after working hours.

When the problem is actually present, here are some coping skills that may prove helpful:

- Use self-talk such as "I can get through this" or "I am not going to buy into this stuff."

- Strongly focus on one aspect of the situation so that other aspects are shut out. For example, in a hostile work environment an individual can concentrate on the particular task and shut out everything else.

- Use breaks as appropriate.

- Understand that "It too shall pass" and that it is "only a matter of time before it will be ended and I will be doing something else."

Restore the Balance

Even though the situation is troublesome for the recovering alcoholic, efforts must be made to restore balance, equilibrium, and emotional stability. These restorative activities usually follow the problem situation. For example, an individual may go for a walk along the river after a hard day at work in order to settle down and relax. The point is that the earlier situation can and will disturb the individual. If steps are not taken to offset these negative effects, the problems will grow and fester leading to a more serious disturbance for the individual.

There are many activities available for restoring the balance. Individuals are encouraged to select those activities that they are familiar with and have some expectation that following the activity, they will become more settled. Clearly, recovering alcoholics should select activities on the basis of their effectiveness in helping the individual to relax and restore balance. Following are some common strategies for helping a person to relax and restore balance:

- Taking a walk

- Working out at the gym

- Gardening

- Listening to music or playing an instrument

- Reading a popular book

- Surfing the Internet

- Shopping

- Relaxation breathing

- Yoga

- Meditation

- Hobbies

- Taking a class

- Other

Seek Support

No Cost or Low Cost Personal Support. Often available at no cost are organized support groups for situations that cause stress and are ongoing problems such as groups for abused women, cancer support groups, bereavement groups, parenting groups, and veteran groups. These groups can be particularly helpful because of the common bonds that are formed through the shared experiences. There are many support groups whose primary purpose is to provide acceptance, fellowship, guidance, and support—such as Alcoholics Anonymous, Al-Anon, Save Our Selves (SOS), and Rational Emotive Behavior Therapy (REBT).

Other No cost Support. Of special importance for an individual who is coping with a problem situation is the support role of a family member, friend, or sponsor. A counselor is a common option as well. It can be easy for an individual to become discouraged with having to deal with a problem situation that does not change. Personal support can help to build up one's resilience, belief in oneself, and persistence in coping with the situation.

Seek Professional Support. In some problem situations it may be highly desirable for an individual to seek professional help such as therapy, or psychological and psychiatric help. This level of support is needed when individuals are dealing with something traumatic such as divorce, mental and emotional crises, death, or chronic sickness in the family. Clearly, for this level of support to be pursued, the individual would need to have the necessary insurance or resources to cover expenses.

Note: This chapter's focus is on autonomous growth. Support groups and personal support persons are necessary in the early stages of recovery—in establishing *beginning sobriety* (Section Two, Chapters 4, 5, and 6). At this juncture, once beginning sobriety has been attained, the recovering alcoholic is in the process of *phasing out* the role of the support groups and support persons in order to work toward *autonomous growth*. The pace of phasing out the level of support will vary from individual to individual. The rule is that it is better to maintain some level of support than to remove support entirely and suffer a relapse.

Checklist and Action Plan for Coping Skills

The following checklist and action plan is intended as a guide for recovering alcoholics to help them to develop and implement coping skills for problem situations that are uncontrollable and unchangeable.

Readers are then encouraged to select which items might best work for them in the *Yes/No* column and then provide a brief description in the *Notes* column of how they intend to use the item, and rating the effectiveness of the strategy after it has been implemented. A blank form is presented in the appendices section, Appendix H: Form 8.4, Checklist and Action plan for Coping Skills, and an example is described in Illustration 8.4.

Chapter Summary

One of the biggest challenges facing individuals after they quit drinking lies in the area of autonomous growth. Alcoholism by definition is a loss of autonomy in that the alcoholic is controlled by alcohol resulting in a very definite dependence (an addiction). However, just because individuals have quit alcohol, this does not mean that they have achieved autonomy in other important areas of their lives. On the contrary, recovering alcoholics most often experience a void or are at a loss after they become sober, even when it comes to making the simplest of decisions, such as whether to go to a meeting or not, to managing their affairs in a timely manner. As alcoholics, they have grown accustomed to living without exercising autonomy in many important areas of their lives. Now that they have quit alcohol, they have to learn, or relearn, how to take charge of their lives.

The approach in this chapter has been that becoming more autonomous means to acquire a set of skills that enable autonomous growth. These skills have been described as taking charge of necessary areas of life, learning how to problem solve, how to overcome procrastination, make decisions and take charge of personal affairs, and how to develop and complete to-do lists in a timely manner. In addition, there are problem situations that may arise which the recovering alcoholic may determine to be uncontrollable and unchangeable. In these situations the individual must learn to develop and implement coping skills. It is assumed that by becoming more autonomous in major life areas the recovering alcoholic will enjoy a richer life free of alcohol.

Background: Chuck is a retired city worker and lives by himself as his wife died a few years back. He has always been a heavy drinker but since he retired and his wife died he has been drinking more and more to the point that he couldn't stop. His doctor told him he needs to quit and recommended a counselor who could help. Chuck followed through and had been able to maintain sobriety now for 4 months. Now that he was sober he found things began to annoy him more. One particular annoyance was the guy in the apartment below who played loud music at night. He concluded that earlier when he was drinking, he was not bothered by the music. Now it really bugged him. He tried talking to the guy and tried turning up his own music. A couple of times he banged a broom on the floor. He put in a complaint to the landlady. Maybe the guy turned the music down some but it still annoyed Chuck. His counselor walked him through the following coping skill steps.

ILLUSTRATION 8.4: Checklist and Action Plan for Coping Skills

Skill	Selection (Underline) Yes or No	Notes
Assessing the problem situation: • Problem is uncontrollable and unchangeable. • Situation can be left.	<u>Yes</u> No Yes <u>No</u>	*Chuck concluded that nothing would change and the landlady said he was the only one complaining. He could not afford to move to another apartment plus the location was right for him for other needs.*
Problem situation accepted	<u>Yes</u> No	*Chuck did not like this deep down but knew it was something he had to live with.*
Manage the moment • Use self-talk • Focus on one aspect of task • Use breaks • Understand "it too shall pass" • Other	<u>Yes</u> No <u>Yes</u> No <u>Yes</u> No <u>Yes</u> No <u>Yes</u> No	*Chuck kept saying to himself, "I can survive this." He got some headphones and listened to his own music. He went for walks and went to the library or coffee shop at times when the guy played his music.*
Restore the balance • Take a walk • Work out at the gym • Gardening • Listen to/play music • Read a popular book/magazine • Surf the net • Shopping • Relaxation breathing • Yoga • Meditation • Hobbies • Take a class • Other	<u>Yes</u> No Yes <u>No</u> Yes <u>No</u> <u>Yes</u> No <u>Yes</u> No Yes <u>No</u> Yes <u>No</u> Yes <u>No</u> Yes <u>No</u> Yes <u>No</u> Yes <u>No</u> Yes <u>No</u> <u>Yes</u> No	*Chuck went for a walk and found the exercise beneficial. He built his own selection of music that he began to appreciate more and more. By going to the library he found he could relax there and get into reading more.* *He had boxes of photos and found great relaxation and memories from sorting the photos and making albums of them. He was then able to show the albums to his daughter which was great for each of them.*

ILLUSTRATION 8.4 *Continued*

ACTION PLAN

Once Chuck realized he was stuck in the situation, he was then able to adapt his routines and activities to cope with the situation. As time went on he was able to include more relaxing activities. Even though the music from the guy below was still a pain, Chuck was able to deal with it and take charge of his own life and interests.

Skills for Cognitive Growth

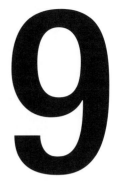

We cannot solve our problems with the same thinking we used when we created them.

— Albert Einstein

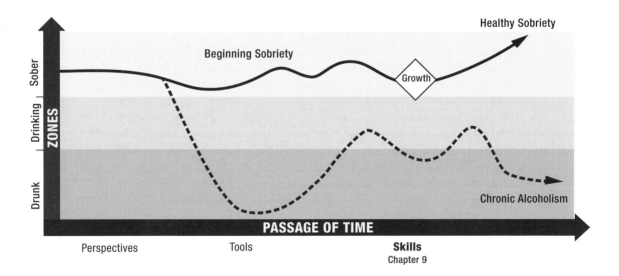

One of the biggest challenges facing recovering alcoholics is to address the need for cognitive growth. When an individual is consumed by alcoholism, a number of deleterious effects arise. It has been well documented in medical research that excessive use of alcohol causes substantial damage to the brain (Bates, Bowden, & Barry, 2002; Harper, 1988; Rosenbloom, Pfefferbaum, & Sullivan, 1995; White, 2003). The ramifications of such brain damage are quite extensive and the negative impact reaches into many aspects of an individual's level of functioning and quality of life. One telling effect of such brain damage from alcoholism lies in the area of *cognitive impairment* such as memory loss and dementia; reduction in attention span; faulty thinking and reasoning processes; and communication issues (Broe et al., 2008; Fein, Bachman, Fisher, & Davenport, 1990). Clearly, deficiencies in these crucial areas of basic mental functioning must lead to diminished or limited lifestyles. Given the recovering alcoholic is motivated to experience an improved life more than sobriety alone, it is imperative that efforts be undertaken to offset these cognitive impairments arising from alcohol abuse.   The purpose of this chapter is to describe interventions that are designed to establish, or re-establish, the cognitive skills that have been weakened through sustained drinking.

The specific cognitive skill areas to be addressed for recovering alcoholics are related to deficits in the areas of: 1. Memory loss, and 2. Faulty thinking patterns.

Memory Loss

It is reasonably safe to say that most everyone by middle age has known somebody who has been afflicted with the memory loss diseases such as dementia and Alzheimer's. The usual communication patterns are no longer present such as recognition of people, especially family and friends, use of names, and recall of events. The afflicted person acts as a stranger or an entirely different person. The effect is disturbing and often devastating for family members and friends. Memory is central to the proper function of an individual for communication, decision making, problem solving, planning, social activities, and so many of life's activities. When the memory faculty is reduced, or destroyed, as in the case of dementia and Alzheimer's, the quality of life for the individual is significantly altered.

Recovering alcoholics also may face this problem of memory loss in varying degrees. Alcoholics and binge drinkers often report that after a certain point while drinking, they lose their memory. They have no recollection of events that occurred after this point is reached. The police and courts are all too familiar with the plea of "I don't remember" following criminal or potential criminal incidents when alcohol is involved. Alcohol-related dementia is called Wernicke-Korsakoff syndrome which is manifest by impaired memory, learning problems, creation of false experiences, and problem-solving difficulties. These effects are believed to be caused by deficiencies of thiamine (vitamin B1). The disease can be prevented with diet and alcohol control along with vitamin supplements.

The extent of the damage to the memory faculty is usually related to the stage of alcoholism reached (Chapter 4). The alcoholic who has been drinking excessively for many years, late stage, will have more memory loss than an early-stage alcoholic simply because more brain damage has occurred in the case of the late-stage alcoholic. Moreover, it is reported that short-term memory loss is more evident during the first few months of abstinence from alcohol compared to the loss experienced by recovering alcoholics with several months or years of abstinence (Fein, et al., 1990).

Recovering alcoholics experience impairments to their memory faculty have significant impact on their day-to-day living. Recovering alcoholics who want to improve the quality of their lives by working toward a sober healthy lifestyle need to address these memory impairments caused by alcoholism. Typically, there are two steps for addressing memory issues: 1. Identify the signs of memory loss, and 2. Take concrete steps to enhance the memory faculty. A checklist and action plan is provided for both of these steps followed by an illustration.

Step 1: Identify the Signs of Memory Loss

The following symptoms for memory loss are typical for individuals recovering from alcoholism, but not necessarily exhaustive or complete. The last item, "Other," is included for those symptoms that may occur for an individual but are not included on this list.

1. **Loss of Recall**. Here the recovering alcoholic has difficulty recalling facts, happenings, and information from past or recent events. Also, parts of something can be remembered but not all of it.

2. **Easily Distracted.** The individuals have great difficulty maintaining a series of thoughts or tracking a conversation. They have difficulty maintaining a flow of conversation in that they get going on a subject then switch to something else. They are very easily distracted and often get stuck in a thought and cannot remember what they wanted to say.

3. **Preoccupation.** Some individuals appear to be preoccupied and it is difficult to engage their attention and certainly difficult to hold their attention.

4. **Short Attention Span.** Related to being easily distracted and preoccupied is the impairment of a short attention span. For example, recovering alcoholics may have difficulty tracking what someone else is saying because they lose concentration or cannot listen for very long. Similarly, they have trouble following the plot in a story in a book, a TV show, or movie.

5. **Difficulty Planning and Following Plans.** A very common and limiting memory impairment is the difficulty an individual has in making plans, developing the concrete steps in a plan, and in following a plan.

6. **Difficulty in Completing Routines.** Once individuals begin a routine, even one that was quite well established earlier on before the onset of serious drinking, such as doing laundry, they stop and start again, do something else, and it is not long before the routine is abandoned.

7. **Misplacing Items.** Some recovering alcoholics become particularly frustrated because they are consistently misplacing needed items such as their car keys, wallets, watches, or cell phones. The problem is exacerbated because they also have great difficulty in retracing their steps and being able to recall when they last used the item. Sometimes individuals are convinced that they left the item in a certain place which is not the case.

8. **Difficulty in Making Conversation.** Since some recovering alcoholics have difficulty with memory recall, they have problems in making conversation. They typically become frustrated with themselves and others because of these difficulties and reach a point where it is better to avoid the social contexts rather than endure the indignation of struggling conversations or interactions.

9. **Forgetting Familiar Routines.** It is common for recovering alcoholics early in recovery to lose track of familiar routines such as getting lost on the way to a friend's house when they have been to the house often or forgetting how to bake certain items. Similarly, they forget the purpose of certain activities such as why they are doing an errand or making a phone call.

Step 2: Take Concrete Steps to Enhance the Memory Faculty

It has been widely established that certain strategies can assist persons with memory problems. These strategies have emerged from research and practices for dealing with issues with the aging process, memory diseases (dementia, Alzheimer's, and Wernicke-Korsakoff syndrome), brain injuries, and persons afflicted with alcoholism. Many of the strategies are also used by very busy people who need assistance to ensure that important responsibilities are dealt with in a timely manner. Recovering alcoholics are encouraged to try certain strategies and determine what works best for them.

1. **Write It Down**. The age-old practice of *write it down* is an effective and easy-to-use strategy for supporting the memory faculty for two reasons. First, writing something down serves as a permanent and visual reminder of a task or responsibility that needs to be addressed. Second, the act of writing an item down helps to register the information with the memory. Most people experience that by writing something down they are more likely to remember the particular item. A common practice for recovering alcoholics is to write notes or messages to themselves to jog their memory. It is most important that a set place is determined for where to put these notes such as a corner of the kitchen counter or a bulletin board. The recovering alcoholic needs to check this location as a daily or regular routine and to remove notes that are out of date.

   Sponsors and support persons for recovering alcoholics typically encourage recovering alcoholics to keep a notebook or diary (physical or electronic) and to use it frequently to write down tasks, responsibilities, activities, perceptions, concerns, and ideas.

   There are many ways a person can write something down, for example: diary, journal, notebook, notepad, index cards, post-it notes. Also many people make use of electronic devices such as a smartphone, PDA, tablet, computer, or iPad. Some recovering alcoholics reported making use of recording devices. Another common strategy is to make use of an erasable whiteboard in the home or a bulletin board.

The notebook or diary serves as a basis for subsequent discussions and review of events. The diary can be kept on one's cell phone, or other device, but if it is not kept in a set place at home, they can lose track of it and become frustrated because they cannot remember where they put it.

2. **Use Visual Cues**. It is helpful for some individuals to use visual cues or prompts to remember things they have to do. For example, they leave some laundry in the hallway to remind them to do the laundry that evening, or they leave an item for recycling item near the door to remind them to put out the garbage in the morning.

3. **Have a Set Place for Frequently Used Items**. One recovering alcoholic said that she had to have a set place for everything she uses. "I always put my car keys and purse on the dressing table, my messages and to-do lists go on the corner of the kitchen counter." She also commented that as time went on she had a set place for almost everything in her home which saves a lot of panic and frustration from trying to find things.

4. **Use Repetition**. Another age-old strategy for memory building is rote practice or repetition. When something is repeated over and over (drill as it is often called), the individual has more chance of retaining the information. Recovering alcoholics can greatly profit by repeating information, asking others to repeat information such as, "What was your name again, please?" or "Where is it that you work?" The rote actions combined with writing information down can make an immeasurable difference in the memory functioning for a recovering alcoholic.

Similarly, it is helpful in communication with others to *paraphrase* what has been communicated. By repeating back what has been said, the recovering alcoholic helps to ensure that what has been communicated has been understood and there is more chance, through the repetition, of remembering what was said.

5.   **Engage in Memory-Based Brain Games**. The memory faculty can be perceived in much the same way as a muscle group. By exercising the muscles, they remain flexible and serve us better. When we do not exercise them, they stiffen up and become injury prone. It is in our best interest to take care of our muscles and do what we can to maintain their proper functioning. Similarly, with memory, we can engage in activities that stimulate the memory or simply keep it working. Or we can vegetate, not engage the memory, and experience ongoing memory loss.

There are many opportunities for recovering alcoholics to exercise their memory faculty. One common strategy is to make use of activities that have been called *memory-based games,* so called because they are designed to stimulate and engage the memory. The games include puzzles, crossword puzzles, board games based on memory such as Trivia Pursuit, Facts and Five, card games, and countless other games that can be purchased, borrowed, or used at agencies or organizations. In addition there are countless memory games available for computers, smartphones, and hand-held devices.

6.   **Establish Routines**. One of the many negative results from alcoholism is that the individuals lose a lot of their daily living routines. They become so consumed by the need to drink that all else becomes of secondary importance. Many of these routines for daily living need to be restored and new ones established such as grocery shopping, house cleaning, preparing for work, managing finances, and taking care of family. Once the recovering alcoholic determines what routines are needed and what they look like, the next step is to practice them over and over until the individuals are quite *fluent* with them. Fluency with routines means that the individual can complete the routine automatically or without thinking. Clearly, if the recovering alcoholic establishes routines and can complete them automatically then there are fewer demands on memory. The activities are wired. In this way responsibilities are much more likely to be completed with minimal dependence on memory.

7.   **Stimulate the Mind.** The mind and the memory are closely linked. By stimulating the mind, individuals are more likely to stay on track or hold their attention in conversations, reading materials, and in entertainment such as movies. There are many ways to stimulate the mind by engaging in high interest activities, hobbies, walks, outings, and visits to centers such

as museums, craft shows, and fairs. Similarly, there are many pencil and paper and electronic activities that stretch the mind including Sudoku and other puzzles. If the person likes to read but cannot handle long books, then choosing short stories or magazine articles of interest will build up a base of attention and concentration. A short attention span can gradually be lengthened by choosing high interest activities of short duration to begin with and systematically engaging with longer duration activities.

8. **Physical Exercise.** Last, but certainly not least, we come to the powerful role of exercise. The all-round benefits of physical exercise have been so well documented over the years that the practice has become standard measure or routine for maintaining health and preventing problems for all age groups. More specifically, Medina (2008) reported research indicating: a. Substantial gains were made in all cognitive areas by individuals who engaged in regular exercise compared to those who did not; b. That risk of general dementia is cut in half for individuals who have participated in regular exercise; and c. That exercise can substantially benefit those who have had various forms of brain damage. In summary, Medina (2008) reported that:

> A lifetime of exercise can result in a sometimes astonishing elevation in cognitive performance, compared with those who are sedentary. Exercisers outperform couch potatoes in test that measure long-term memory, reasoning, attention, problem solving, and even so-called fluid intelligence tests" (p. 14).

Checklist and Action Plan for Memory Loss

The following checklist and action plan is intended as a guide for recovering alcoholics to help them to identify areas where they may be experiencing memory loss and to select strategies for enhancing their memory skills.

Recovering alcoholics are encouraged to underline which items might apply to them regarding memory loss in Step 1, *Yes/No* column and then provide a brief description or comment in the *Notes* column. Items selected as *Yes* are totaled and entered in the Results for Step 1 section. Higher scores denote more effort and time is needed to use strategies to assist memory recovery. In Step 2, the recovering alcoholic selects strategies that might work for them. Comments for the selected strategies are written in the *Notes* column (where the items may be obtained). In the action plan section, the individuals write down the specifics of how they propose to use the strategies (such as what time of day, location, and with whom they may be engaging in the activity).

A blank form for this checklist presented in the appendices section, Appendix I: Form 9.1, Checklist and Action Plan for Memory Loss, and an example is described in Illustration 9.1.

Background: Anne is a 43-year-old 5th grade teacher with just over 11 months of sobriety following her 2nd attendance at a local treatment center. Her principal told her that she needed to be sober at school to keep her job. She is not a member of any recovery program but she has as mentor friend, Karen, a senior teacher, who is a recovering alcoholic with 15 years sobriety. Anne expressed concern about her lack of progress mentally in that she gets muddled a lot, is quite forgetful, and gets into difficulties and problems with other faculty members. She told Karen that "I seem to think just the way I did when I was drinking and get into the same difficulties with my co-workers." Karen suggested that they meet weekly after school and begin with this checklist and action plan.

ILLUSTRATION 9.1: Checklist and Action Plan for Memory Loss

Step 1: Identify the Signs of Memory Loss	Selection (Underline) Yes or No	Notes
1. Loss of recall	Yes <u>No</u>	*Not at work*
2. Easily distracted	<u>Yes</u> No	*Not when I am teaching, but when I am alone or at home I have this problem.*
3. Preoccupation	<u>Yes</u> No	*This happens at school and home. Kids tell me it is hard to get my attention at times.*
4. Short attention span	Yes <u>No</u>	*Again, I am OK at school but not at home.*
5. Difficulty planning and following plans	<u>Yes</u> No	*I can follow them once they are made, but I have trouble making plans.*
6. Difficulty in completing routines	Yes <u>No</u>	*Not that I know. However, I will keep an eye on this one.*
7. Misplacing items	<u>Yes</u> No	*This is a nightmare—keys, purse, my kids assignments. I even forget where I parked my car sometimes.*

ILLUSTRATION 9.1 *Continued*

8. Difficulty in making conversation	<u>Yes</u> No	*I have trouble making conversation at lunch. I end up just sitting there saying nothing but answering a question when asked.*
9. Forgetting familiar routines	<u>Yes</u> No	*I go shopping and forget what I need even for one or two items.*
10. Other	Yes <u>No</u>	*Not at work*
Results for Step 1 Total number of *Yes* Scores __**6**__		
A. 6 or more *Yes* items selected	<u>Yes</u> No	<u>Significant problems</u> *6 is a pretty high score.*
B. 3–5 *Yes* items selected	Yes <u>No</u>	Some problems
C. 1–2 *Yes* items selected	Yes <u>No</u>	Minimal problems
Step 2: Take Concrete Steps to Enhance the Memory Faculty		
1. Write it down	<u>Yes</u> No	*I carry a notebook with me, review it often, and chat with Karen about it.*
2. Use visual cues	Yes <u>No</u>	
3. Have set place for frequently used items	<u>Yes</u> No	*I put my car keys and purse on the nightstand all the time and started to have a set place in the house for most things.*
4. Use repetition	<u>Yes</u> No	*I repeat names and important things to myself a couple of times.*
5. Engage in memory-based brain games	<u>Yes</u> No	*This need is met at school, but I am going to add a game or two to my phone.*
6. Establish routines	<u>Yes</u> No	*I make a to-do list each evening for the next day and put it in my notebook.*
7. Stimulate the mind	Yes <u>No</u>	*Again, this need is met teaching. I do read a little and watch TV—more to relax.*
8. Physical exercise	<u>Yes</u> No	*I get some exercise when I have to walk but will walk each evening when I get home. Karen is very adamant that I do more exercise and get a fixed routine.*
9. Other	Yes <u>No</u>	

ILLUSTRATION 9.1 *Continued*

ACTION PLAN (Combining Steps 1 and 2)

1. *I meet with Karen after school on Thursdays (neither of us have meetings then).*

2. *Karen suggested to work on memory issues first and to tackle getting along with others and social skills later on.*

3. *Designate a set place at home for essentials (car keys, etc.) and reorganize the kitchen so that each item has a set place. Change a few things in the classroom with Karen's suggestions—student assignment box, organizers for supplies and materials.*

4. *Sit down after dinner and make a to-do list for the next day in my notebook and check off items for the current day.*

5. *Call Karen or text each evening after to-do list has been made for brief report (Karen's suggestion).*

6. *Either watch movies I like or read my favorite classics for the hour or so before I go to bed.*

Faulty Thinking Patterns

One of the most devastating and long-term harmful effects of alcoholism is the substantial limitations incurred on the mind or intellect. Specifically, the impact on the way the individual *thinks*—the thinking patterns. It is as if alcoholics begin to wear blinders so that their perceptions of the world, events, interactions, and life itself becomes quite distorted and has one focus—themselves. One explanation is alcoholism causes individuals to be consumed with the need to drink and that everything else begins to pale into insignificance. Thinking skills such as judgments, problem solving, interpretations, inferences, and conclusions are basically shelved or restricted to areas that concern maintaining the drinking habit and dealing with or manipulating the repercussions from drinking excessively. These thinking skills that are limited to supporting the habit of alcoholism are labeled and are quite pervasive. The thinking skills have been impaired.

The recovering alcoholic, accustomed to using thinking skills to support the habit of alcoholism now has the daunting challenge of using these skills in a life free of alcohol. The situation is analogous to an individual whose writing has been limited to sending out short memos to the staff who now has the responsibility for writing short stories for a magazine. The experience of writing memos is nowhere near adequate to prepare this individual to write quality articles of length for a magazine. Or, an individual is used to supervising one or two people in a job and now has a new job that requires supervising 50 people. The original experience is of limited use in preparing the person for the new position. Moreover, the individual may have learned practices that worked with the original job but are actually obstructive in the new job.

The recovering alcoholic is initially equipped with a set of thinking skills that is essentially destructive and limited to supporting the habit of alcoholism. Now the individual is faced with having to use these skills for a life without alcohol, which is not a good fit. The individual must now re-tool and learn a new set of thinking skills for healthy sobriety.

It was reported that a recovering alcoholic asked at a meeting, "What is alcoholic thinking?" The response was very telling and represents the theme of this section:

> Alcoholism isn't so much a drinking problem as it is a thinking problem. Once I quit drinking, the next hurdle is to change my thinking. (Sober Recovery Community, 2009)

The issue for the alcoholic is that the destructive thinking skills that were operating during alcoholism are now operating during sobriety. The challenge for the alcoholic is to acknowledge the situation and take the necessary steps to build and learn a new set of constructive thinking skills that will enable the individual to live a richer quality of life. There are two steps for developing a new set of thinking skills: 1. Identify the destructive thinking patterns, and 2. Take concrete steps to build constructive thinking skills. A checklist and action plan is provided for each of these steps, followed by an illustration.

Step 1: Identify the Destructive Thinking Patterns

Destructive thinking patterns are those practices that an individual uses while an alcoholic. These patterns need to be identified in early sobriety and replaced by constructive thinking skills. It might be noted that this list of erroneous thinking patterns was raised in conjunction with the *dry drunk syndrome* described in Chapter 7 where individuals who become sober still carry the same limited or negative ways of operating as when they were alcoholics. The following list represents common faulty thinking practices for recovering alcoholics.

Inability to Make Decisions. The recovering alcoholic often has trouble making the simplest of decisions such as whether to get the groceries now or later. With bigger decisions it is not uncommon for the individual to freeze or procrastinate. Decision making is hard.

Grandiosity. The individuals have an exaggerated or unrealistic assessment of their own abilities and importance. They know how to talk big but when it comes to action, they disappear. They are also prone to exaggeration and to embellishing accounts of events with credible-sounding but untrue details.

Judgmentalism. This behavior is particularly annoying and causes social problems. The individual is constantly negative about other people's actions and frequently critical of their decisions and performance.

Intolerance. Here the individual reacts quite negatively to other people's mistakes or efforts and also shows prejudice when faced with differences or diversity.

Manipulative. The individuals know what they want and use others to obtain their desires. They put a lot of pressure on their friends, relatives, and contacts and become very demanding in order to get what they want.

Self-Centered. It is very evident that the individuals are only concerned with themselves and display little or no concern regarding the feelings and needs of others. They often display tunnel vision where they only have one limited view of things and that view is typically centered on and limited to themselves.

Dishonest. Denial and lack of honesty have been a way of life. Lying, cheating, stealing, making false promises, making up stories, and distorting reality for their benefit are common behaviors.

Impulsivity and Instant Gratification. Alcoholics live in the present moment, so immediate gratification is the norm. They have to have what they want immediately and are driven to act without thinking things through.

False Attribution. Individuals are very quick to blame others for problems or put interpretation on circumstances such as "You did this on purpose."

Victim-Entitlement Cycle. Recovering alcoholics often feel very sorry for themselves (which is probably a major reason they became alcoholics). They readily assume the victim role and as a result believe they are entitled to many things such as support, opportunities, special consideration, and hand-outs.

Obsessing. Recovering alcoholics are typically in a void once they quit drinking. Some fill the void with a single thought. They obsess about a certain thing or obsess about two or three items going from one to the other. Oftentimes they perseverate on a problem ("I lost my job" or "I don't like my apartment") and they will not let the problem go (nor will they address a solution).

Step 2: Build Constructive Thinking Skills

It is particularly important that the recovering alcoholic not become discouraged when faced with these destructive thinking patterns. The changes will take time, effort, and support. The recovering alcoholic must believe that an individual can *learn* constructive thinking skills by using the following well documented effective strategies. Some of these recommendations were identified as crucial strategies for obtaining beginning sobriety (such as going to meetings, and obtaining a sponsor). These same strategies can be adapted to enable the recovering alcoholic to attain the critical thinking skills needed for attaining healthy sobriety.

1. **Learn from Meetings.** Recovering alcoholics, especially during early sobriety, are *strongly encouraged* to attend meetings on a regular basis. These meetings provide support, show the individual how others deal with issues, provide feedback and encouragement from the participants, and insight or understanding of the process of recovery (as noted in Chapters 5 and 6). Once the person has become sober, the next step is to use the meeting as an opportunity to learn skills shared by participants at the meeting on the subject of constructive thinking skills. Typically, there is a broad range of meetings which focus on different topics and needs. The recovering alcoholic, with some effort, can usually find a meeting that addresses their needs, especially in the area of personal skill development.

2. **Learn from a Sponsor or Support Person.** Once again the role of a sponsor or personal support person is strongly recommended in the process for

recovering alcoholics. It is very common to change sponsors as the needs of the recovering alcoholic change. Initially, the focus is in quitting drinking and a particular sponsor may have solid skills in providing support to address cravings and initial needs (Chapters 5 and 6). However, once the recovering alcoholic has maintained sobriety for some time, it usually becomes necessary to shift to a sponsor who has more experience or background in skill-building for personal growth (autonomous, cognitive, social, and emotional). An important responsibility of the sponsor in this role is to challenge the recovering alcoholic when faulty thinking patterns are observed and to review options that are constructive. In addition, the sponsor needs to support, encourage, and acknowledge choices the recovering alcoholic makes using constructive thinking patterns. The role of the sponsor in this stage of cognitive growth can be particularly helpful for the recovering alcoholic.

3. **Learn from Professional Help.** In more severe cases where the recovering alcoholic becomes embroiled with faulty thinking and cannot rise out of these patterns, professional assistance may be needed. These individuals need the expertise of counselors, therapists, or psychologists to help them unravel the operating destructive thinking patterns and build replacement strategies for constructive thinking.

4. **Learn from Journaling and Reflecting.** Some individuals profit greatly from using a notebook or journal for identifying their thinking patterns. By noting their thoughts, decisions, and outcomes on a regular basis, they are in a position to examine and reflect on the way they are operating and the progress they may or may not be having. A journal used in conjunction with sponsor support, or professional service, is a very effective way for establishing and maintaining constructive thinking patterns.

5. **Learn from Significant People.** In some cases friends, relatives, church leaders, workmates, and supervisors can provide important feedback to a recovering alcoholic when they see behavior related to faulty thinking. There is nothing like a close friend saying something like, "Golly. You were very harsh with Sarah today. What were you thinking?" These situations are usually informal and not that frequent. However, they may serve as a wake up-call to a recovering alcoholic that can set in motion efforts to change their thinking.

6. **Learn from Classes.** A formal approach to addressing faulty thinking habits is to attend classes. Self-help and service-related classes are available at times through university and community colleges, churches, hospitals, and services agencies. These classes center on helpful topics such as anger management, conflict resolution, and responsible decision making. Sometimes a guest speaker who is an authority, researcher, or author on one of these topics, may be presenting locally or may be accessed online.

7. **Reject Negative Thinking.** Faulty thinking is basically negative thinking and, is to be avoided. In some cases when recovering alcoholics consistently use faulty thinking patterns and do not build appropriate constructive thinking patterns, they can fall into the trap of *pervasive negative thinking*. In this situation they become inundated or consumed with negative thoughts which can readily lead to troublesome negative feelings (such as fears, anxieties, and depression). This topic of emotional issues arising from sustained negative thinking will be addressed in Chapter 11: Skills for Emotional Growth.

Checklist and Action Plan for Faulty Thinking Patterns

The checklist and action plan for this section is intended as a guide for recovering alcoholics to help them to identify patterns of faulty thinking and select strategies for building and maintaining constructive thinking skills.

Recovering alcoholics are to select which items might apply to them. In Step 1, items related to destructive thinking patterns are underlined as appropriate in the *Yes/No* column followed by a brief description or comment in the *Notes* column. Items selected as Yes are totaled and entered in the Results column. The higher the score denotes more effort and time is needed to use strategies to assist with developing constructive thinking skills. In Step 2, strategies are selected which might work for the individual in developing constructive thinking skills. Comments for the selected strategies are noted as appropriate, such as where the strategies may be accessed and arranged. In the action plan section, the individuals write down the specifics of how they propose to use the strategies such as what time of day, location, and with whom they may be engaging in the activity.

A blank form is presented in the appendices section, Appendix J: Form 9.2, Checklist and Action Plan for Faulty Thinking, and an example is described in Illustration 9.2.

Background: Ben is a 28-year-old who has been sober for 3 years. He attends a local church and has a close relationship with the pastor. There is a men's group at the church which meets regularly on a variety of topics from fundraising, to work parties, and Bible studies. He is aware of a number of the members who are recovering alcoholics and some who drink heavily. He works as a security guard at a local mall. His concern is "I still think crazy, even after quitting drinking for 3 years. I don't know sometimes which is real and what I have made up. I still find I react to what others say and do and they get annoyed with me. I get tired of others telling me I am arrogant and that I don't listen to them and they sometimes mock what I have to say. To top it off, a good friend took me aside and told me that he thought I was 'being a jerk' at the meetings. I spoke to my pastor and he mentioned that he has seen other members have problems long after they quit drinking. He thought that alcoholics develop bad thinking patterns and need to learn new ones. He offered to work with me on this and use this checklist and action plan."

ILLUSTRATION 9.2: Checklist and Action Plan for Faulty Thinking Patterns

Step 1: Identify the Destructive Thinking Patterns	Selection (Underline) Yes or No	Notes
1. Inability to make decisions	<u>Yes</u> No	*At home but not at work. My girlfriend calls me Mr. Waffle.*
2. Grandiosity	<u>Yes</u> No	*My good friend tells me I come across like this to others.*
3. Judgmentalism	<u>Yes</u> No	*I see people saying a lot of stupid stuff which really annoys me.*
4. Intolerance	<u>Yes</u> No	*I rarely agree with what others say and get annoyed when they don't follow my ideas.*
5. Manipulative	<u>Yes</u> No	*I don't see this but others tell me I am.*
6. Self-Centered	<u>Yes</u> No	*Again, it is others that see me as this.*
7. Dishonest	Yes <u>No</u>	*I believe I am doing the right thing. I am not deliberately dishonest.*
8. Impulsivity and instant gratification	<u>Yes</u> No	*Yep. That's me to a tee. I want it and want it now.*
9. False attribution	<u>Yes</u> No	*Yes, I see intention behind a lot of what people do and blame them.*
10. Victim-entitlement cycle	Yes <u>No</u>	*I get angry but don't think I play the victim role. (I see others doing this all the time!)*
11. Obsessing	<u>Yes</u> No	*Yep, when I get get caught up with something I have a hard time letting go.*
12. Other	Yes <u>No</u>	

ILLUSTRATION 9.2 *Continued*

Results for Step 1 Total number of *Yes* Scores **9**	Selection (Underline)	Notes
A. 6 or more *Yes* items selected	<u>Yes</u> No	<u>Significant problems</u> *My score of 9 Yes items means I need to address my faulty thinking and get a solid plan.*
B. 3–5 *Yes* items selected	Yes <u>No</u>	Some problems
C. 1–2 *Yes* items selected	Yes <u>No</u>	Minimal problems
Step 2: Build Constructive Thinking Skills		
1. Learn from meetings	<u>Yes</u> No	*A buddy tells me his group has great sharing beyond just being sober. I will go to this group.*
2. Learn from sponsor or support person	<u>Yes</u> No	*My pastor offered to serve as a sponsor/counselor. He knows what I need so I am seeing him once a week.*
3. Learn from professional help	Yes <u>No</u>	*I'll see how it goes with my pastor.*
4. Learn from journaling and reflecting	<u>Yes</u> No	*Definitely. I will journal and take it to the visits with my pastor.*
5. Learn from significant people	<u>Yes</u> No	*I have identified 2-3 good friends and will ask their opinion from time to time on how I am doing.*
6. Learn from classes	Yes <u>No</u>	*Not yet, but might consider it if the other steps don't work.*
7. Reject negative thinking	<u>Yes</u> No	*Yes, I definitely need help here and will address it with my pastor.*
8. Other	<u>Yes</u> No	*I like reading, so will find some books on positive thinking.*

ILLUSTRATION 9.2 *Continued*

ACTION PLAN (Combining Steps 1 and 2)

1. Attend new AA meeting recommended by a friend.

2. Visit with my pastor once a week—Wednesday evenings is best for each of us. Check in daily with a phone call, email, or text.

3. Note down events in my journal that make me mad with other people and track my negative thinking about them.

4. Visit with my close friends and chat about my behavior in meetings.

5. Find some good books on positive thinking.

Chapter Summary

Alcoholics, because of the very nature of their addiction develop a series of coping skills that are designed to primarily support their habit of excessive drinking. As a result, they develop an array of thinking patterns that end up being quite destructive and limiting. Consequently, when they quit drinking they experience significantly impaired cognitive skills of reasoning, problem solving, and general interpretation of reality. Recovering alcoholics face the choice of leading a life of sobriety with impaired cognitive skills or taking measures to rebuild these skills so that they not only remain sober but can also experience cognitive growth and enjoy life more fully. In effect they need to replace destructive thinking patterns developed in their days of alcoholism with constructive thinking skills for a healthy life of sobriety.

A critical area of cognitive impairment for excessive alcohol use is damage to memory from relatively low impact on short-term memory to serious memory loss issues known as Wernicke-Korsakoff syndrome. Common signs of memory loss and effective strategies for memory improvement are identified followed by a checklist and action plan for individuals to develop their own memory recovery plan.

A second major cognitive impairment from excessive alcohol use is identified as faulty thinking. Two steps are described for addressing this problem. The first step involves identifying faulty thinking patterns that individuals may be presently using that were in use when they were alcoholics. A list of these faulty thinking patterns is described and a checklist is presented for the recovering alcoholics to determine the current status of their faulty thinking patterns. The second step is to use time-tested and effective strategies for replacing these destructive thinking patterns with constructive cognitive skills. A number of these strategies are described and listed. The recovering alcoholics are encouraged to select from this list the strategies that might be a good fit for them and proceed to implement the procedures.

While cognitive impairments typically occur following a period of alcoholism, these problems can be reversed in varying degrees through the use of well-documented practices. It is in the recovering alcoholics' best interest to take definite steps to use these methods with the goal of establishing a healthy lifestyle.

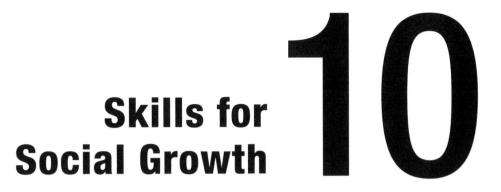

Skills for
Social Growth

10

*Real success is not on the stage, but off the stage as a human being,
and how you get along with your fellow man.*

— Sammy Davis, Jr.

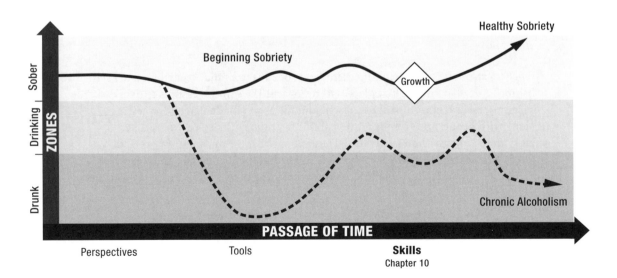

It has been long established that social norms and cultural practices play a key role in establishing alcoholism. For example, the pressure to drink at certain events such as celebrations for graduation, birthdays, weddings, birth of newborns, end-of-the-year parties, beginning-of-the-year parties, weekly get-togethers, and so it goes. In some cultures it is a badge of honor to be a big drinker, for example, "Sonny sure can hold his drink. He can drink anyone under the table," is a typical comment. College parties, especially fraternities, are notorious for beer-drinking games and competitions. Many cultures have the practice of buying a round or sometimes called having "shout." In these cases an individual is expected to take a turn to buy everyone in the group a drink which not only puts pressure on everyone to have several drinks but also to drink at the same rate as the group. This pressure to drink at social events often gets a person started with the practice of drinking regularly and, in some cases, heavily, which can set the stage for alcoholism. This factor will also be addressed in Chapter 12 under the subject of relapses.

Another aspect of social factors related to alcoholism is the deep-seated need people have to belong, be with friends, be appreciated, and get along with others. Some individuals feel quite inadequate in meeting these needs because they are shy, feel inhibited in groups, become anxious that they may make inappropriate comments, react negatively to what others say, or act in odd or antisocial ways. In these cases, some individuals discover that alcohol helps them overcome these fears and anxieties and that they can actually enjoy themselves with others after they have had a few drinks. In general, they learn that deficiencies in social skills can be attenuated through alcohol use. Again, the stage is set for some of these individuals to become alcoholics.

Once an alcoholic quits drinking then these social factors that contributed to establishing alcoholism in the first place will resurface. The same pressures to drink at certain social events will still be present and the social inadequacies for getting along with people and feeling comfortable in a group will also re-emerge, perhaps even more strongly than in the initial situations. In addition, some recovering alcoholics realize after they have become sober that these good social times when drinking were really very shallow. As one recovering alcoholic shared at a meeting:

> I found that I wasn't drinking with my friends. I was drinking by them.

The purpose of Chapter 10 is to address the topic of *social growth*. The basic assumption is that while the recovering alcoholic has made great gains in maintaining sobriety, there are some entrenched needs that have not been met and one of these centers on developing adequate *social connections* at work, in the community, and at home. The idea is that once a person becomes sober and takes the necessary steps to meet social needs, a richer and healthier lifestyle will ensue.

The specific areas of social growth addressed are: 1. Understanding social competence, 2. Negative effects of social deficiencies, 3. Indicators of social competence and social deficiencies, 4. Strategies for developing social competence, and 5. Checklist and action plan.

Understanding Social Competence

Recovering alcoholics often experience significant difficulties in developing and maintaining satisfactory interpersonal relationships; communicating with other people (especially people outside of support groups); feeling comfortable in a group; knowing the right thing to say and what not to say; engaging in enjoyable conversations; and in achieving social acceptance from peers, coworkers, and others. In a word, many recovering alcoholics are typically quite deficient in *social competence*.

Definition of Social Competence

Social competence is a very broad term describing a person's ability to get along with and to make appropriate responses to other people in various circumstances. Social competence involves some kind of response or action from one individual to another individual or individuals. The response can be verbal, written, a transfer of an object such as a gift or reminder, or a gesture. This response may affect the other person or persons either in positive, negative, or neutral ways.

There are four key dimensions or properties of social competence: 1. Critical discriminations followed by appropriate responses, 2. Awareness of how a response may be received, 3. Judgment on the appropriateness of the response, and 4. An emphasis on the response being acceptable rather than perfect.

1. **Critical Discriminations Followed by Appropriate Responses**
   This is the key really. An individual needs to be able to read the situation and based on that reading make a response that is appropriate. For example, if a person appears to be upset, then the individual's response to that person would be more cautious and supportive than if, say, the person is laughing loudly and having a good time. Social graces or skills mostly rest with a person's ability to know *what to say when*.

2. **Awareness of How a Response May Be Received**
   In a similar way, socially competent people are aware of how their response is likely to be received. For example, if an individual picks up that a person is sensitive about weight or the quality of their work, then the individual would be careful about alluding to weight or performance issues. Or, if a person barely knows another person, then it is best to avoid personal issues because it is not known how the comments will be received.

3. **Judgment on the Appropriateness of the Response**
   Social competence basically is a judgment on the *outcome* of how responses are likely to be received by another individual or a group of individuals. If the responses are accepted by the individual, the responses are said to be socially appropriate. If the responses are frowned upon or received unfavorably, then the responses are socially inappropriate.

4. **An Emphasis on the Response Being Acceptable Rather Than Perfect**
   Social competence is not to be equated with perfection. Rather, the standard is that the responses need to be in the *acceptable range*. In this way social competence can be attained by most people who are motivated to learn the skills and put them to work in their daily lives.

Another way of understanding social competence is to examine its opposite or antonym—*socially deficient behavior*. Socially deficient behavior refers to that cluster of human behaviors where individuals respond to others in a way that has a negative impact. These behaviors have the effect of alienating other people, hurting their feelings, frustrating them, causing them harm or embarrassment, and losing their respect. Social competence, by contrast, enables a person to reach others and obtain their respect and friendship.

In Box 10.1 two vignettes are presented showing positive and negative examples of social competence.

BOX 10.1: Positive and Negative Examples of Social Competence

VIGNETTE 1

Sarah was sitting at a table in a coffee shop by herself with a paper and coffee cup in front of her. She was staring at the table, with her hands under her chin, and looking quite serious and subdued. Belinda, a recovering alcoholic comes into the coffee shop notices Sarah and heads over to her.

Negative Example	Positive Example
Belinda says in an upbeat manner, "Hi Sarah. Great seeing you. You'll never guess what happened last night. Let me get a cup of coffee and I'll tell you all about it." She heads off to get her coffee.	*Belinda notices Sarah is looking flat and stands near her and pauses. Sarah looks at her. Belinda says, "Hi Sarah. Good to see you. Would you like some company?" Sarah nods her head. Belinda says, "Thanks. Let me get some coffee and I'll be right back."*

Comments

In the negative example, Belinda is totally unaware of the stress Sarah is showing. She just barges in and wants to tell Sarah of some event from the night before. Belinda is not attending to Sarah at all and is only focused on herself and may end up worsening the situation for Sarah.

In the positive example, Belinda notices Sarah is looking down and subdued, approaches her quietly and does not invade her space and waits for recognition from Sarah. Belinda in this case is attending to Sarah, recognizes she may be upset, respects her space, gets permission to join her, comes across as supportive and may end up making the situation better for Sarah.

VIGNETTE 2

A community-based outreach group was in a heavy discussion on how to help a family. Some wanted to get right in, build some things for them, and help them with cash for a short term. Others thought the family was malingering and needed to help itself. One shouted, "I thought we are Christians." Another shouted back, "Being Christian does not mean enabling slackers." Jon, a recovering alcoholic, came into the meeting late.

Negative Example	Positive Example
Jon could clearly feel the tension and thought he should shift the focus. He said, "Let me tell my story. It might help." He then proceeded to describe in detail how he became an alcoholic, all the problems it caused, how he became sober, took care of his family, and now has been sober for two years.	*Jon could clearly feel the tension and thought he should sit quiet for a while to get more of a feel of what was happening. The shouting continued for some time, Jon suggested that they might adjourn, pick this issue up at the next meeting, and in the meantime some of the group might go visit the family and see if they could get a joint plan, with concrete steps for the family and the group.*

> **BOX 10.1** *Continued*
>
> ### Comments
>
> In the negative example, Jon read there was a problem but he jumped in to fix it with his own story. He probably annoyed everyone by taking over after being late and trying to solve the problem by going off in another direction. Also, he probably really annoyed the group by taking up their time by running his story and presuming they would be interested at this moment. In subsequent meetings Jon would probably be cut off.
>
> In the positive example, Jon read the tension and knew his place. It was not his business after coming in late and missing the early information to tell them what to do. Rather, he waited patiently, came across as trying to defuse the situation and solve the problem. The group probably wanted to end the hostilities so Jon's suggestion gave them a way out and the plan to followup was sensible. In contrast with the negative example, Jon's judgment would have been respected and in future meetings the group would listen to him.

Attaining Social Competence

There is no question that a recovering alcoholic can remain sober without addressing social concerns. However, we would argue that social competence is needed to attain a satisfying *quality of life*. Moreover, it is logical to expect that once a higher quality of life is experienced, the recovering alcoholic is less likely to turn to alcohol. So an important question arises for the recovering alcoholic, "Am I socially competent?" or "Is social competence something that I really need to work on?"

Given that there are substantial social pressures to drink alcohol and that many alcoholics turned to drinking in the first place to meet social needs or to overcome social difficulties, it is very important for recovering alcoholics to examine their level of social competence. The first step is to evaluate whether or not the recovering alcoholic needs a social competence intervention. The most direct indicator to answer this question is whether or not the recovering alcoholic is experiencing a degree of pain, discomfort, or significant limitations from the effects of social deficiencies. If this is the case, then the individual would profit from an intervention designed to improve social competence.

Typically, most recovering alcoholics have social skill impairments because of the effects of sustained use of alcohol and antisocial practices used during this period. There are three steps in addressing social competence for recovering alcoholics: 1. Assess the negative impact of social deficiencies, 2. Pinpoint specific social deficiencies, and 3. Develop an intervention for social competence.

Step 1: Assess the Negative Impact of Social Deficiencies

One way to assess the extent of social impairments and whether or not a social competence intervention is needed is to carefully review the impact social deficiencies have had in crucial areas of the recovering alcoholics life. Five impact areas of social deficiencies are described followed by a rating scale.

Impact Areas of Social Deficiencies

1. **Impact on Employment.** Many recovering alcoholics report that they have either lost their jobs or have difficulty keeping a job. One reason for these difficulties is the ability to get along with their co-workers or supervisors. Inability to get along with others is usually ranked as one of the major reasons for a person being fired. The work environment itself, specifically difficulties in getting along with others, is cited as one of the most common reasons for people walking off a job (Fontana, 1994; Simerson & McCormick, 2003). Interpersonal relationships play a critical role for a person in being hired, maintaining a job, and obtaining job satisfaction.

2. **Effect on Relationship**s. Alcoholics have often reported how relationships have been threatened or ruined through excessive drinking. Similarly recovering alcoholics report problems with existing relationships at the level of communicating adequately and being aware of the needs of others. Simply put, the recovering alcoholic often does not have the social skills to maintain and develop personal relationships.

   Other recovering alcoholics find difficulty in establishing new relationships and in keeping them once they are underway. One recovering alcoholic pointed out that he had been an alcoholic since high school and that he had never learned how to ask someone out for a date. Now he is thirty-three with four years sobriety, and he still struggles with knowing what to say to someone just to go to a movie. He finds he would sooner stay home, or go by himself, rather than become embarrassed with fumbling for what to say to someone for a date or an outing. Others have reported that they are comfortable in speaking in a group, but when it comes to being with someone on one-to-one, they really struggle with what to say.

3. **Alienation.** Recovering alcoholics often get a sense that no one wants to be around them. Their antisocial and self-centered behavior makes it difficult for people to want to visit with them, spend time with them, or engage them in conversation. Some recovering alcoholics begin to feel a sense of rejection. This kind of rejection is usually not blatant (for example, they might not be directly confronted about their behavior). Rather, the feedback is more subtle in that people move away from them, find excuses to leave and not return, and that no one is actually approaching them for conversation. These feelings were not that important when they were drinking because it was always relatively easy to find someone to drink with—just walk into a bar. However, now that the individual has quit drinking, there is more of a need to be around people.

    In many cases this need, especially in early sobriety, is met by participating in the fellowship offered by support groups such as Alcoholics Anonymous. In these contexts an individual's antisocial behavior is understood and tolerated. In addition, constructive feedback is sometimes provided which helps individuals change their behavior (at least to remove some of the rougher edges). Other recovering individuals, later in sobriety, often want to expand their social competence to be able to participate in more mainstream groups and to be accepted without this feeling of alienation.

4. **Experience of Loneliness.** Everyone experiences loneliness at some time, especially following difficult circumstances such as the death of a spouse, break-up of a relationship, loss of job, or relocation to a new city. These situations are usually of a temporary nature. However, in the case of the recovering alcoholic, the loneliness arises from an inability to make satisfying friendships and relationships and are more long-term in duration. They have to learn how to relate to people in new ways now that they do not have "a drink in hand." Quite often the recovering alcoholic makes overtures to connect with people that fail. They are often not even aware of why their efforts fail. Some experience direct rejection because they may have been too forceful, too insensitive to the situation, too talkative, especially about topics that interest them but have little interest to others, perhaps become too personal too quickly, and many have difficulty correctly reading situations and say or do something inappropriate.

    In some cases, recovering alcoholics feel that the only people they can talk to are other recovering alcoholics—their kindred souls. While this contact is very important, especially early in sobriety, it may not be sufficient later on in sobriety for some individuals. One reason is that some recovering alcoholics feel the need for more in-depth or more personal conversations than what they experience in early sobriety. For example, one recovering alcoholic mentioned to his sponsor, "You know, sometimes when I am talking with some of my recovering alcoholic buddies it is not like a dialogue, it is more like crossed monologues!"

5. **Limited Problem Solving Skills.** It is standard practice for most people when they have a problem to call someone or talk to someone about how to deal with the situation. The need may be just to vent, which is helpful for some, or to explore options for a solution. In the case on many recovering alcoholics this option may be limited because they may not have that many people to turn to. In some cases, the only people they can turn to are other recovering alcoholics. While this can helpful, and is not to be criticized, it can be limiting for some recovering alcoholics. Some individuals have great difficulty describing a problem. In addition, recovering alcoholics are often sidetracked by issues that are only peripherally related to the problem. Consequently, when they discuss or report a problem they cannot give sufficient information for their friend, sponsor, or support person to help them address the problem.

Rating Scale for Impact of Social Deficiencies

It is very predictable that recovering alcoholics will have deficiency in social skills. The rating scale, Form 10.1 (Appendix K) is designed to help the recovering alcoholic determine the extent to which the effects of social deficiencies have impacted their lives and to determine the need for a social competence intervention. Recovering alcoholics are encouraged to examine each item and assess the impact the item is having on their lives on a scale of 0 to 2 where a rating of zero denotes no impact at all, 1 represents some impact, and a rating of 2 denotes serious impact. Comments or explanations for the particular rating selected are indicated in the *Notes* column. The results are tallied and the recommendation is that if an individual scores a total of 5 or more, then a social competence intervention is needed.

A blank form is presented in the appendices section, Appendix K: Form 10.1, Rating Scale for Impact of Social Deficiencies, and an example is described in Illustration 10.1.

Background: Jim, a 42-year-old chronic alcoholic, had been drinking since he was 12 and had been involved with the legal system since his early years. He was incarcerated for driving under the influence in a hit-and-run accident leaving someone seriously injured. He had a steady girlfriend for 3 years. Upon release, he lived in an Oxford house (supported living center for recovering alcoholics), for one year and presently he is living in an apartment and has a job at a local supermarket. He is still on probation and meets with his probation officer every other week. After 12 months of maintaining sobriety and keeping his job, in a meeting with his P.O. he said, "You know I am just a sober ex-con. I just don't know how to be with people, I don't get it. I sit at home with my brother and the only conversations are about work stuff. I feel people are avoiding me. There has to be more to life than this." Jim's P.O. said, "Let's try to see what is going on and have you fill out this form."

ILLUSTRATION 10.1: Rating Scale for Impact of Social Deficiencies

Crucial Life Areas	Rating of Impact (Underline) 0—No impact 1—Some impact 2—Serious impact	Notes
1. Employment (At risk? Written up? Warned?)	<u>0</u> 1 2	*I can do the job. I don't get along with co-workers. They talk to me about work stuff otherwise they avoid me like the plague.*
2. Relationships (Have friends? Go to gatherings? Meet?)	0 1 <u>2</u>	*I have tried to make friends, but people seem to pull away from me no matter how hard I try. I tried to connect with my former girlfriend but she is uncertain or wary.*
3. Alienation (Rejected? Left out?)	0 <u>1</u> 2	*I sure feel alone or pushed aside if that's what it means.*
4. Loneliness (Feel the pain or pinch? Brood? Worry about being alone?)	0 1 <u>2</u>	*Absolutely. I feel lonely at home and on the weekends. Strange, but even at work when I am with people I still feel lonely.*
5. Problem solving (Fix things? Talk things through?)	0 1 <u>2</u>	*I try to solve problems and want to solve them but am not successful.*
6. Other (for example, Awareness)	0 1 <u>2</u>	*I was never aware of these problems when I was drinking.*
Results Total Score **9**	Selection	Notes
A. Score of 6 or more	<u>Yes</u> No	<u>Full social competence intervention needed</u> *My sponsor will work with me on a plan.*
B. Score between 2 and 5	Yes <u>No</u>	Some intervention needed
C. Score less than 2	Yes <u>No</u>	No intervention needed
DECISION		

Social competence intervention is needed. Proceed with Step 2: Pinpont specific social skill deficiencies, and Step 3: Develop an Intervention Plan for Social Competence.

Step 2: Pinpoint Specific Social Deficiencies

If a recovering alcoholic experiences any of the negative impact from social deficiencies identified in Form 10.1 to a marked degree (score 2 or more), then steps need to be taken to build social competence. Key questions for the recovering alcoholic become "What am I doing that leads to these negative predicaments?" and "What do others do that I don't do?" In other words, what exactly are the social skills or competencies other people have that the recovering alcoholic lacks that may be causing these negative effects? Conversely, what skills need to be developed to enable the recovering alcoholic to experience a higher quality of life that social competence can generate?

Box 10.2 lists identifies common indicators of social competence that are considered to be standard or acceptable. The approach taken is to describe each social indicator of social competence in conjunction with its polar opposite—social deficiency. The indicator of social competence is the skill that the recovering alcoholic needs to build and implement and the social deficiency is one that may already be present and needs to change. In Box 10.2 common indicators of social competence are described in the column on the left and the corresponding social deficiency is described in the column on the right.

BOX 10.2: Indicators of Social Competence and Corresponding Social Deficiencies

Social Competence	Social Deficiency
Honesty: Is straightforward in communicating and working with people. There are no hidden agendas or manipulations.	**Dishonesty:** Communication is devious and manipulative. Lying and cheating is common.
Empathetic: Shows concern and support for others. Is aware when things are not right for others and communicates this awareness.	**Insensitive:** Does not notice or care about difficulties others may be facing. Main concern is self and others are not important.
Remorseful: Displays concern when errors are made. Shows ownership with problems and intent to learn from mistakes.	**Unrepentant:** Is not bothered by mistakes and does not show concern or ownership. Does not show willingness to learn from mistakes.
Peaceful: Generally is not looking for trouble and prefers problems to be solved amicably.	**Aggressive:** Seems to be looking for trouble and thrives on opportunities to confront and engage in altercations.
Problem solves: Is solution oriented when problems arise. Energy goes to solving the problem.	**Blames others:** Main focus is always to blame others, protect self from blame, avoid ownership, and avoid finding solutions.
Calm: Generally responds to issues and concerns in a calm and unruffled manner.	**Angry and irritable:** First reaction is usually anger and irritability.
Controlled: Knows it is important to think things through and not to react too quickly. Responds to issues in a planned manner.	**Impulsive:** Reacts very quickly to situations. Wants to respond immediately and usually without planning.
Responsible: Is aware of danger or negative impact to self and others and is cautious about safety concerns.	**Irresponsibile:** Is reckless, likes to take risks, and ignores safety concerns for others and self.
Responsive: Is willing to act as soon as reasonable when situations demand it, especially issues for others.	**Non-responsive:** Usually is not aware or oblivious to the concerns of others so is perceived as non-responsive. Also heavily focused on self so that needs of others are not recognized.
Attentive to others: Attends to others, listens to what they say and waits for the right moment to respond, responds appropriately, and communicates interest and concern.	**Self-centered:** Does not show interest in others, interrupts them, and directs the conversation to own needs or stories.
Communicates: Is able to make own points or needs known. Can communicate so that they are understood. Speaks to concerns in a timely manner.	**Miscommunicates:** Has poor ability to make own needs known or understood. Often leaves the other person wondering what was said or meant or with the wrong information. Allows concerns to fester and communicates too late.
Follows procedures: Is aware of rules and procedures and follows them in general.	**Non-complies:** Resists directions and procedures and is driven to follow own rules and procedures.
Sexually appropriates: Has appropriate intimate relationships with other people built on trust and consent.	**Promiscuous:** Uses sex and intimacy as a tool for own needs or to exploit and use others. In some cases individuals use promiscuity as a way to gain attention.

Rating Scale for Social Competency

A social competency rating scale is presented in Form 10.2 (Appendix L) based on the indicators of social competence and social deficiencies described above. The intent is for recovering alcoholics to determine the extent to which these specific indicators of social competence and social deficiencies are presently operating in their lives. The idea is that recovering alcoholics examine each indicator and its polar opposite as a continuum and determines where they see themselves in this continuum. The scale is designed as a two-tail or two-direction measure with the indicator for social competence pointing to the left (to the descriptors in the column for social competence) and the corresponding indicator for social deficiency pointing to the right (to the descriptors in the column for social deficiency). A score of zero, in the middle of the continuum, means that neither the social competency nor the social deficiency is operating to any discernible extent; a score of 1 means that the competency or deficiency is somewhat operating; and a 2 means that the competency or deficiency is definitely operating. Recovering alcoholics are encouraged to underline the score (0, 1, or 2) and direction (toward the social competency direction to the left or social deficiency to the right) that best meets their assessment. Comments or explanations for the particular rating selected are indicated in the Notes column. The items scored with a 2 or 1 in the social deficiency direction or 0 are identified for intervention.

A blank form is presented in the appendices section, Appendix L: Form 10.2, Rating Scale for Social Competence, and an example is described in Illustration 10.2.

Background: Since Jim scored 9 on the previous Rating Scale for Impact of Social Seficiencies (Form 10.1) indicating that he is in serious need of a social competence intervention. His P.O. discussed the results with him. Jim agreed to pursue the social competence training, "Whatever it takes," he said. His P.O. said that the next step is to see how Jim rates with the major social competencies. To this end, the P.O. helped Jim to complete this form.

ILLUSTRATION 10.2: Rating Scale for Social Competence

Social Competency	Rating (Underline) 0—Not applicable 1—Somewhat applicable 2—Very applicable	Social Deficiency	Notes
1. Honesty	2 1 0 **1 2**	1. Dishonesty	When I lie it is more to protect myself so I don't get into trouble or have people think less of me.
2. Empathetic	2 1 0 **1 2**	2. Insensitive	I guess I don't show empathy or understanding. Something I never worried about when I was drinking.
3. Remorseful	**2** 1 0 **1 2**	3. Unrepentant	You betcha. That's why I am doing this. I want to do better with people.
4. Peaceful	**2 1** 0 **1 2**	4. Aggressive	I don't want trouble. But it finds me and I react.
5. Problem solves	2 1 0 **1 2**	5. Blames others	Again I want to fix things but don't know how to I guess.
6. Calm	**2** 1 **0 1 2**	6. Angry & irritable	I can go either way so I put myself in the middle.
7. Controlled	**2 1** 0 **1 2**	7. Impulsive	I am better at this but have a ways to go. I know when I am being impulsive.
8. Responsible	2 **1** 0 1 2	8. Irresponsible	I sure learned in prison to be careful but not sure how I will do now I am out. I am cautious.
9. Responsive	2 1 0 **1 2**	9. Non-responsive	You know I'd like to be responsive to people but when I try to be I seem to drive a wedge between us rather than connect.
10. Attentive to others	2 1 0 **1 2**	10. Self-centered	For years I have been number 1 and that is hard to change. I'd like to.
11. Communicates	2 1 **0 1 2**	11. Miscommunicates	I am in the middle here. I communicate with my P.O., was fine in jail, and with alcoholics when I was drinking. But now at work and with other people I don't do well at all.
12. Follows procedures	**2** 1 0 **1 2**	12. Non-complies	I am a good worker and can follow rules and didn't have trouble in jail with following rules.
13. Sexually appropriate	2 1 **0 1 2**	13. Promiscuous	I really don't know where I stand here as I haven't had a lady friend for years.
	1 2 Danger Zone		

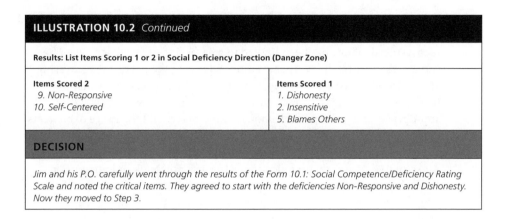

ILLUSTRATION 10.2 *Continued*

Results: List Items Scoring 1 or 2 in Social Deficiency Direction (Danger Zone)	
Items Scored 2 9. Non-Responsive 10. Self-Centered	**Items Scored 1** 1. Dishonesty 2. Insensitive 5. Blames Others

DECISION

Jim and his P.O. carefully went through the results of the Form 10.1: Social Competence/Deficiency Rating Scale and noted the critical items. They agreed to start with the deficiencies Non-Responsive and Dishonesty. Now they moved to Step 3.

Step 3: Develop an Intervention for Social Competence

The previous two forms, Form 10.1 and Form 10.2, provide the recovering alcoholic information on whether or not social deficiencies have impacted negatively in crucial areas of their lives and which specific social deficiencies are pertinent. The next step is to develop a checklist and action plan for an intervention to develop social competence in needed areas arising from the results from Forms 10.1 and 10.2.

A major theme in this book is that a recovering alcoholic can learn the skills necessary to live a sober, fruitful and healthy life. In this case, recovering alcoholics may need to address the subject of social competence. Many recovering alcoholics may have experienced the harmful effects of social competence deficiencies described earlier in this chapter and have identified the presence of social deficiencies in their dealings with others. The next step is to systematically learn or strengthen the skills for social competence needed for successful, ongoing, interpersonal relationships. These skills would then be applied to the areas of concern that were identified in the social competence rating scales (Form 10.2 and Illustration 10.2).

The main strategies for learning and developing new skills, in this case for social competence, center on: 1. Active reflection, 2. Ongoing feedback from a support person, 3. Attendance at meetings and related social gatherings, 4. Engaging in service work, 5. Modeling from significant persons, 6. Stepping out and taking measured risks, 7. Understanding and maintaining relationships, 8. Seeking professional help, and 9. Using self-help instruction.

1. **Active Reflection.** There is no substitute for individuals taking a close look at how they conducted themselves on specific occasions. For example, a recovering alcoholic has been invited to a gathering of friends to celebrate someone's 40th birthday. That evening, following the party, the recovering alcoholic reflects on the evening, how it went, the conversations that were involved, the feelings that may have arisen during the evening, whether appropriate or inappropriate responses were made, and the range of contacts made.

    A useful tool to assist with reflection is to use a notebook or journal. For example, following a gathering a person would sit down, with a cup of tea maybe, and note down anything of significance that may have occurred. Sometimes it is helpful to read back through other similar gatherings and examine how these situations were handled compared to the current entry. In this way an individual can assess progress, recurring strengths or weaknesses. If recurring weaknesses (indicators of social deficiencies) are noted, then the individual needs to develop a more concrete plan to address the problem or seek help.

2. **Ongoing Feedback from a Support Person.** Once again the support person, sponsor, close friend, or church member, can be of invaluable assistance in helping a recovering alcoholic address social competence needs. If these meetings are conducted on a regular basis, it usually does not take very long for the support person to recognize signs of social deficiencies in their sponsee. For example, any hostile and resentful feelings toward others, if present, will readily surface in meetings. Similarly, the sponsors will spot very early in the meetings whether the recovering alcoholics are attentive, listening, and are empathetic or focused primarily on themselves and their own needs.

    It is imperative for the support person to use the meetings as a critical growth opportunity for the recovering alcoholic. To this end the support person must be straightforward and directly challenge the recovering alcoholic when instances of antisocial behavior emerge. Direct feedback is most important. As someone at a meeting commented, "A good sponsor must make you mad at times, if you want to grow up." The recovering alcoholic is also encouraged to make use of the notebook or journal at meetings and to share what has been noted and reflected upon.

3. **Attendance at Meetings and Related Social Gatherings.** It is typically recommended that recovering alcoholics attend meetings to assist them with processing their journey from alcoholism to their recovery. It is generally thought to be of great assistance to hear other recovering alcoholics share their stories which can serve to validate others. Recovering alcoholics can learn from meetings that they are not such a "loser," "odd-ball," or "bad person." Moreover, they can receive inspiration and enlightenment from how others have successfully addressed common problems.

    Of particular importance is the focus on *acceptance* at these meetings. A recovering alcoholic does not have to work hard to be accepted by this group, as might be the case in other social gatherings. The mere fact that the recovering alcoholic shows up is sufficient to be accepted, as Alcoholics Anonymous (2008) unequivocally states in their 3rd Tradition: "The only requirement for AA membership is the desire to quit drinking" (p. 139).

    Another dimension that can be particularly helpful in the development of social competence is attendance at social activities sponsored by recovering alcoholic support groups. These activities give the recovering alcoholic an opportunity to get to know others, at a more social level, who are on a similar recovery journey, "kindred souls" so to speak. At these gatherings the recovering alcoholic has the opportunity to exhibit social competence (or deficiencies) in a relatively safe environment (safe because of the basic acceptance among recovering alcoholics who are trying to remain sober).

4. **Engaging in Service Work.** One of the surest ways of connecting with people, attending to the needs of others, and looking beyond the needs of self is to undertake service work. The Twelfth Step in Alcoholics Anonymous is very clear on this important function for effective recovery. There are many opportunities for service work in communities such as the Salvation Army, St. Vincent de Paul, schools, libraries, hospitals, and specific service organizations. Recovering alcoholics are encouraged to look around for service opportunities where they can bring their specialized skills as appropriate or, for that matter, volunteer for any service activities where they are basically comfortable. Some recovering alcoholics have felt more comfortable in volunteering for service work in the company of another recovering alcoholic or a friend. This situation makes the situation somewhat safer for them and provides an opportunity to share the experiences.

5. **Modeling from Significant Persons**. It has been well established in research and literature that a predominant way children learn social skills is through modeling—by following the example of important people in their lives such as parents, older siblings, relatives, and teachers (McGinnis & Goldstein, 2003; Patterson & Forgatch, 2005). Similarly, adults, in this case recovering alcoholics, can hone social skills by following the example of adults they respect. For example, the recovering alcoholic might observe the way a coworker manages a conflict or watch how a good friend moves around at a gathering to chat briefly to everyone, or watch the positive interactions between another recovering alcoholic and his girlfriend.

    By observing examples of social competence in other respected persons, recovering alcoholics are also looking beyond themselves which helps them to become less self-centered and more tuned into others. Again the recovering alcoholic is strongly encouraged to write down in their journal their observations, reactions, thoughts, and feelings, for reflection and discussion with their support person.

6. **Stepping Out and Taking Measured Risks.** It is possible for a person to have attained many years of sobriety but to have lived a very sheltered or protected existence. One need recovering alcoholics have is to remain sober, which of course is paramount, and the other is the need for a deeper or more meaningful social existence. On the one hand there is no way the individuals want to put their sobriety at risk, but they also ask, "Is there more to life than just being sober?" The challenge becomes how to maintain sobriety and yet to step out a little and expand one's social life. At one level, recovering alcoholics may have fears that they will jeopardize their sobriety if they go to parties and other social gatherings where alcohol is part of the function. At another level, recovering alcoholics may fear rejection or social failures in reaching out to people. They understand that they have impairments regarding social competence and worry they might put their foot in it, annoy someone, or become annoyed themselves. Some have deep fears regarding dating simply because they are not sure how to ask someone out or what to talk about when they are out. In effect there is *risk involved* when individuals try to expand their social life. A guiding rule for expanding one's social life is to take *measured steps to minimize the risks*. For example, a recovering alcoholic reported that she went to four AA meetings per week. Now she goes to three AA meetings and attends a book reading club. The book reading club has replaced one of her AA meetings (she still attends the other

three AA meetings). Another recovering alcoholic indicated that he always attended the recovering alcoholic social functions. He now goes to most of them but also goes to events sponsored by his church and work place. The key to avoiding big problems in stepping out is to do it gradually by slowly introducing other activities and in keeping some of the original activities. In this way individuals can control the rate of expansion of their social activities and not get burned if things do not work out the way they intended or hoped they would.

7. **Understanding and Maintaining Relationships.** One reason that recovering alcoholics run into difficulties with making friends, keeping friends, dating, and in making conversation in general, is that they do not have a good understanding of the concept of *levels of relationships*. For example, if a recovering alcoholic is talking to someone for perhaps only the second time, it would be inappropriate to share something very personal. This would most likely be off-putting to the other person. Whereas, if the person was a very dear long-time friend, it would be quite appropriate to share something of a personal nature. A socially competent person understands the concept of levels of relationships and the corresponding ways of interacting at each of these levels. The recovering alcoholic, who has trouble making and maintaining friends may need to study and apply the following information on levels of relationships.

The literature on interpersonal relationships address several levels ranging from three to seven (Burton & Dimbleby, 2006; Kelly, M., 2007; Greenfield, 1984). For the purposes of this book, four levels of relationships will be described to give the recovering alcoholic the basic concepts and general directions for application: a. Casual, b. Companionship, c. Personal, and d. Exclusive.

> *Casual Relationships.* This level is the most basic and covers relationships at an acquaintance level. The conversations would be simply about events, facts, the weather, sports results, general topics and could be called small talk. The response about such a relationship would be "I know that person."

> *Companionship Relationships.* At this level the communication is centered *in common interests.* They share information of their experience and knowledge about certain hobbies or activities, such as fishing, coin collections, landscape, a sport team, or building

and construction. They might attend outings together that focus on this common interest. The exchanges, apart from these specific common interests, would mostly be centered on small talk. The response about such a relationship would be "He is my fishing buddy" or "She is my guitar connection."

Personal Relationships. Here the relationship is much deeper and has been sustained over a longer period of time. This relationship speaks to a friendship level where personal or private information can be shared. The person feels comfortable sharing things that are of concern and even embarrassment because there is a deep sense of trust. The response about such a relationship would be "He (or she) is a very dear friend."

Exclusive Relationships. In this relationship one person is committed to the other in a long-term manner and no other person can fill this particular role such as in marriage or as significant partners. The level of sharing covers the full range from small talk to highly personal matters. Moreover, the relationship can accommodate periods of little communication as each person is quite comfortable just being in the other's presence. Physical and sexual intimacy is usually an integral part of this level. The response about such a person would be "She (or he) is my partner or wife or husband" or "I am seeing him (or her)" or "This is my soul mate."

The overall point is that there are levels of relationships and that these levels dictate the kind of information that is exchanged. In addition, it might be helpful for the recovering alcoholic to understand that the levels of relationship also function as a progression. That is, a relationship can start out as casual and upon further contact move to *companion* and then to *personal* and *exclusive*. It is also suggested that recovering alcoholics could use this information to determine the status of the relationships they presently have. It is assumed that quality of life requires relationships at least to the level of *companionship* and, ideally, to the *personal* and, in some cases, to the *exclusive* levels.

8.   **Addressing Sexual Relationships**. Sexual activity can occur between consenting adults without the expectation that a relationship may or may not develop. Sexual activity can also occur at any level of a relationship from *casual* through to *exclusive*.

Recovering alcoholics can experience a full array of sexually related problems not only when they were drinking but also once they quit. There may have been reported cases insensitivity, disregard, or even abuse towards spouses, partners, or close friends when the individuals were under the influence of alcohol related to sexual activity (reported in Chapter 1). Consequently, these issues may still need to be addressed even when the person has quit drinking. In addition, the other party in these relationships may also need assistance in working through these situations as well.

Other problems have also been identified: Some alcoholics report changes in their sexual activity as a result of drinking and then quitting. For example, sex drive may be altered in either direction—from being less active or more active. Recovering alcoholics, especially long term alcoholics, have indicated that they are very unsure of themselves regarding sexual activity after they have quit alcohol. As one thirty-eight-year-old recovering alcoholic said, "I feel like a teenager when it comes to sex. I am very nervous and unsure of myself." Finally, a big danger facing some alcoholics is that some may use sexual activity by becoming promiscuous to fill the void created from alcohol withdrawal.

It is clear that sexual relationship issues can be quite serious and need to be addressed. We strongly recommend that recovering alcoholics who experience problems in this area seek professional help from counselors or family therapists for themselves and for their spouses, partners, and friends as needed. Also, a variety of free information on these topics is available online from the National Institute on Alcohol Abuse and Alcoholism , NIAAA, (such as *Alcohol Problems in Intimate Relationships: Identification and Intervention*, http://pubs.niaaa.nih.gov/publications/niaaa-guide/NIAAA_AAMF_%20Final.pdf).

9. **Seeking Professional Help.** In some cases it may be necessary for the recovering alcoholic to seek advice and ongoing direction from a professional such as a counselor, therapist, social worker, psychologist, or psychiatrist. This option is limited to those who may have insurance or who can afford the costs. However, if accessible, professional guidance can certainly help recovering alcoholics unravel their social inhibitions and deficiencies and take measures toward attaining social competence.

10. **Using Self-Help Instruction.** Some recovering alcoholics may respond quite favorably to self-help programs. These programs require a certain amount of self-starter aptitude and especially the need for accurate and honest self-appraisals.

Self-help programs for developing social competence can be found in the media of books, CDs, DVDs, and online courses and curricula. Examples of self-help programs are presented in Box 10.3: Sample Self-Help Programs for Building Social Competence.

BOX 10.3: Sample Self-Help Programs for Building Social Competence

Books

Malouf, J. M., & Schutte, N. S., (2007). *Activities to Enhance Social, Emotional, and Problem-Solving skills: Seventy-Six Activities That Teach Children, Adolescents, and Adults Skills Crucial to Success in Life.* Springfield, IL: Charles Thomas.

Cyster, E. (2008). *Teach Yourself Etiquette and Modern Manners* (Teach Yourself: Relationships and Self-Help). Blacklick, OH: McGraw-Hill.

DVDs

Coulter, D., Coulter, D., & Coulter, J. (2005). *Manners for the Real World: Basic Social Skills.* Winston-Salem, NC: Coulter Video.

Fox, S. (2002). *Etiquette survival: Dining and Social Skills for Adults and Teens.* Los Gatos, CA: Etiquette Survival.

Online Courses and Curricula

Elliott, R. (2001). *6 Key Social Skills.* www.self-confidence.co.uk/articles/6-key-social-skills/

Kelly, A. (2007). *Social Skills and Communication Consultancy.* www.alexkelly.biz/

Checklist and Action Plan for Social Growth

Appendix M: Form 10.3, Checklist and Action Plan for Developing Social Competence, provides the recovering alcoholic with a list of sound strategies designed to teach and establish social competence. Recovering alcoholics are encouraged to examine each strategy to determine which ones may be workable or not for them by underlining a *Yes* or *No* in the *Yes/No* column. In addition, brief remarks or comments can be made as appropriate in the *Notes* column. In the action plan section, the individuals write down the specifics of how they propose to use the strategies such as what time of day, location, and with whom they may be engaging in the activity. A blank form is presented in Appendix M: Form 10.3, Checklist and Action Plan for Developing Social Competence, and an example is described in Illustration 10.3.

Jim and his P.O. selected *dishonesty* and *lack of responsivenss* as the target competencies for thir intervention. Jim's P.O. explained each of the strategies, and with Jim they identified which ones might be most workable for Jim and built an action plan.

ILLUSTRATION 10.3: Checklist and Action Plan for Developing Social Competence

Strategies for Developing Social Competence	Selection (Underline) Yes or No	Notes
1. Active reflection	<u>Yes</u> No	*I will use a journal and note especially areas of being responsive and attentive to others.*
2. Ongoing feedback from support person	<u>Yes</u> No	*My P.O. and I will meet each week and walk through how I have been doing with social interactions at work and home and discuss my journal entries.*
3. Attendance at meetings and related social gatherings	<u>Yes</u> No	*I will develop a regular schedule of attendance at AA meetings (twice a week) and attend my work social gatherings even if just for a while, attend birthday gatherings, celebrations and so on.*
4. Engaging in service work	Yes <u>No</u>	*Will do later on.*
5. Modeling from significant persons	Yes <u>No</u>	*I will try to watch some respected people at work and see what they do to get along with workmates and discuss this with my P.O.*
6. Stepping out and taking measured risks	Yes <u>No</u>	*Not yet.*

ILLUSTRATION 10.3 *Continued*		
7. Understanding and maintaining relationships	<u>Yes</u> No	*I need to understand more about relationships—read more, discuss more with Jim and then test the waters myself.*
8. Addressing sexual relationships	<u>Yes</u> No	*If I wasn't abusive to my recent girlfriend I was certainly inconsiderate.*
9. Using self-help instruction	Yes <u>No</u>	*Not yet.*
10. Seeking professional help	Yes <u>No</u>	*I feel I have the help I need.*

ACTION PLAN

I have told myself I want to succeed with this effort to build my social competence. I have met all my parole responsibilities and have remained sober. Now I want to have a better social life. To do this I am committed to the following:

1. Keep a daily journal and note especially social interactions throughout the day and efforts I make.

2. Meet with my P.O. each Wednesday at 5 pm and come prepared to discuss my week, especially in regard to efforts, results, exchanges etc, on my targeted social competencies.

3. Attend the Monday and Thursday AA meetings at 7:15 pm.

4. Attend any work social gatherings at work for birthdays and other celebrations.

5. Pay attention to the way respected people at work operate.

6. Study the topic of relationships more and discuss the information with my P.O.

7. Monitor and expand my plan with my P.O. as I progress.

8. I will get professional help with sexual relationships once I am further along in this plan.

Chapter Summary

Social factors have played a key role not only in why certain individuals become alcoholics in the first place, but also in the quality of life of individuals after they become sober. Recovering alcoholics, while they have made commendable efforts to quit alcohol and become sober, still experience voids in their lives. One of these voids is the limited, or in some cases barely-existent, social life. At the heart of the problem is the recovering alcoholics' lack of social competence.

Social competence is that skill which enables people to communicate effectively, understand where each other is coming from and make appropriate responses for given situations, and to establish and maintain fruitful and healthy relationships. Recovering alcoholics are often deficient in this area of social competence which can have serious repercussions for the individual's life in crucial areas such as with employment, home life, and levels of relationships. A rating scale is provided to help individuals assess whether key areas in their lives are impacted by social deficiencies.

There are a wide range of indicators for social competence. A list of specific indicators for social competence and its opposites, social deficiencies, is provided. A rating scale to determine the presence of each social competence indicator and its opposite is provided to help recovering alcoholics identify which indicators may be operating in their lives at the present moment.

The final section of this chapter is centered on describing strategies for assisting recovering alcoholics to build the necessary social competencies that may be lacking in their lives. A checklist and action plan is presented to enable the recovering alcoholic to undertake steps to implement workable strategies and acquire a deeper level of social competence. The overall assumption is that individuals, by using these strategies, will learn the skills necessary for a fuller and healthier sober lifestyle.

Skills for Emotional Growth

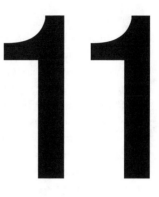

A little kingdom I possess, where thoughts and feelings dwell;
And very hard the task I find of governing it well.

– Louisa May Alcott

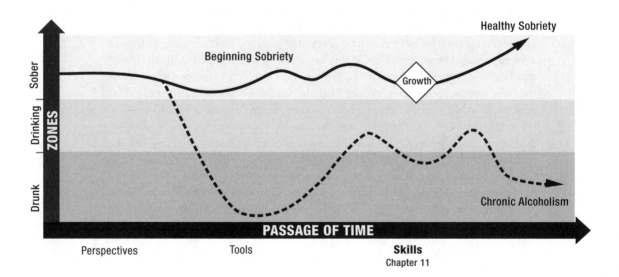

There is no question that emotions or feelings play a powerful role in human behavior, and we are all familiar with the patterns of behavior that are influenced by particular emotions. For example, individuals who are sad and depressed are likely to be subdued and withdrawn. Other individuals who are, instead, very angry can see this anger set the stage for confrontation and fighting. Or, a person who is over-joyful and exceedingly happy may become careless with details or even reckless. Similarly, we are familiar with situations where crowd behavior escalates to violence; where patrons at a concert or public event become unruly; or a protest march where violence erupts between the participants and the crowd or police. A common response to these situations is that "Their emotions got the better of them."

The purpose of this chapter is to address the role emotions play in the lives of recovering alcoholics, in particular to focus on the specific impact alcoholism has had on an individual's emotions and implications for healthy sobriety for the recovering alcoholic. The core assumption is that the recovering alcoholic typically needs to take deliberate measures to attain *emotional growth.*

The first three components, skills for autonomous growth, cognitive growth, and social growth were described in Chapters 8, 9, and 10 respectively and these skills need to be maintained. The fourth component, skills for emotional growth, is addressed in this chapter. The reason emotional growth is presented as the fourth component of personal growth in this section (following autonomous, cognitive, and social growth) is that emotions often arise and become unmanageable from lack of skills in these three earlier-presented areas. For example, a person may be experiencing great anxiety at work because the planned restructuring will cause a lot of personal problems. Now, if this same person has learned skills to be more autonomous, to speak up and make known what may be of concern (Chapter 8), then the worrisome issues are more likely to be addressed. Similarly, individuals may panic over certain situations because there are no apparent solutions. Again, if these individuals have taken measures to develop cognitive skills, to use reason and problem-solving skills (Chapter 9), these situations may be resolved and not lead to panic. Finally, persons who are shy and inhibited may display emotions of fear when it comes to participating in a group activity. However, if these individuals have become more proficient with social competence and have learned how to interact more effectively (Chapter 10), then the feelings of fear may not arise in group situations. The basic assumption is that emotional growth is facilitated by growth in *autonomous, cognitive,* and *social* skill areas.

To recap, developing emotional growth begins with the following strategies:

- Sustained sobriety

- Autonomous growth

- Cognitive growth

- Social growth

The topics addressed in this section include: 1. Understanding emotions, 2. Cycle of emotions, 3. The impact of alcoholism on emotions, 4. General strategies for managing emotions, 5. Specific steps for managing emotions, and 6. Checklist and action plan.

Understanding Emotions

Emotions and their various nuances are known as feelings, sentiments, moods, sensitivities, arousal, and reactions. Most people usually have no trouble knowing what emotions are whether they are experiencing them themselves or seeing them in other people. For example, most people can tell when they are sad, angry, or happy and have no trouble recognizing the same emotions in other people. Yet when we try to define emotions, or try to understand how emotions operate, we run into many complexities which have been a subject of research and debate for many years (Goleman, 1995; McKee, Boyatz, & Johnston, 2008).

Understanding emotions is not a simple undertaking. The challenge in this book is to provide recovering alcoholics with a working understanding of how emotions operate in their lives and especially how these emotions can be managed. In this section, information is provided to give recovering alcoholics a relatively simple understanding of emotions by describing: a. Key characteristics of emotions, b. The classifications of emotions, and c. Emotions as cyclical.

Key Characteristics of Emotions

The following characteristics are considered to be central to understanding emotions and their role in healthy sobriety for the recovering alcoholic.

Physical expressions. Emotions are manifest in a person by physical and physiological responses. For example, persons who are experiencing the emotion of fear may tremble and perspire. Individuals who are in a state of anger may begin to shout and grimace, talk fast, and walk fast. With some people, facial expressions are often a tell-tale sign that certain emotions are presently operating.

Complex interactions. Emotions have often been defined in terms of complex interactions between the environment, an individual's personal history, the brain, physiology, senses, and chemicals in the body. Such interactions are difficult to understand and are the subject of ongoing research. For this book it is sufficient to say that emotions are a function of environment, neurological, and physiological interactions.

Triggering. Typically, emotions are triggered or aroused by some environmental event or thought. For example, a driver could cut someone off in traffic triggering anger for the person cut off (environmental event). Or, a person could be having some coffee and reflect on an interaction with an acquaintance that makes the reflector tremble and become fearful. This acquaintance had previously made serious threats and the mere thought of the person generates fear.

Range of emotions. Most individuals experience a full range of emotions from being happy to sad, joyful to concerned, calm to being upset. Emotions in many cases can change almost immediately. An individual can be feeling quite calm and relaxed then the appearance of another person can turn the emotions from calm to resentful. Similarly, an individual can be cruising quite happily at work and then demands come to complete some tasks immediately which cause anxiety for the person. The experience of a range of emotions is normal.

Emotional states or moods. Some individuals become consumed by certain emotions to the extent that they operate in basically a permanent emotional state or mood. For example, one individual is always angry and can never relax. The anger can lead to ongoing angry behavior (such as arguing, fighting, threatening, abuse, and intolerance).The person is on edge so that anger becomes a way of life. Other individuals can be so consumed by anxiety and depression to the extent that they give up on life and become suicidal. The ideal, of course, is that people are relatively stable in a moderate range of emotional states. However, individuals who experience a more extreme range of emotions or whose more permanent emotional state is mostly at the extreme levels typically need professional help. For example, people who have bipolar disorders are particularly vulnerable to alcoholism because the effects from alcohol consumption can induce a leveling out of emotions. These persons definitely need medical and professional help.

Interplay between thoughts and emotions. The relationship between thoughts and emotions is very much like the chicken and the egg connection. Which came first? It is common experience for emotions to lead to thoughts and for thoughts to lead to emotions. For example, an individual has the thought of wondering what time it is and looks at a clock. Then there is the sudden realization the individual will be late which brings about an emotion of panic through the thought of being late. Another individual may experience the emotion of sadness which generates thoughts on why the person may be sad. The person thinks about having been wronged at work, which gives rise to more sadness and resentment. What we do know is that there is a reciprocal relationship between the emotions and thoughts which has very important implications for defusing and managing emotions (discussed more fully in the strategies section of this chapter).

Motivators of behavior. Emotions play a crucial role in motivating behavior. If a person is angry, that person may exhibit aggressive behavior toward others. If another person is sad or depressed, then this person may decline an invitation to a party. Individuals' decisions can be determined by how they are feeling or what emotions are present at the particular time. Clearly, there can be serious repercussions when important decisions are made based on emotions only, such as in the heat of the moment or when a person feels down and out.

Reason and emotions. There also exists a critical interplay between reason and emotions when it comes to decision making. In most cases, the desirable approach is for individuals to use reason over emotions for important decisions and for responding to challenging situations. Unfortunately, emotions typically rise to the surface first, preceding and overriding reason. The person may feel envious or resentful immediately in a situation which could bring about a negative response, worsening the situation. However, if the person is able to pause, think the matter through, and then act there is more likelihood of a better response. Individuals are constantly challenged when faced with difficult situations to carefully balance emotions with reason.

Gut feelings. While emotions often can dictate behavior as a first response, which can be problematic, there is a definite place for deep-seated or gut feelings when making important decisions. For example, an individual has strong feelings about a situation and comes up with some options using reason. In trying to determine which option is best, a common strategy is to ask "What does your gut feeling tell you?" or "When you boil it all down, how do you really feel about it?" Individuals have found it very helpful in decision making to recognize immediate emotions, use reason to determine options, and then use gut feelings to direct or validate the final decision.

Changing emotions. A very important characteristic of emotions central to this book is whether or not emotions can be lessened (defused or attenuated) and whether emotions can be built up or strengthened. For example, if a person feels strong resentment, are there things that can be done to reduce the intensity of the resentment or even make it go away? Or, if individuals do not experience much joy in their lives, can their lives become more joyful? In other words can *emotions be managed?* The authors believe the answer is an emphatic yes and information will be presented to this end later in this chapter in the sections on strategies and steps for changing emotions.

Emotions in themselves are not value laden. A very strong position is this book is that emotions *in themselves* are neutral—they are neither bad nor good. For example, some individuals may feel the emotion of resentment and consider this feeling as a fault or character defect. No, we take the position that emotions are neither faults nor virtues. Rather, they are simply part of one's makeup. The value-laden dimension comes into play when the person acts on the emotion. For example, if the person feels envy toward someone and then goes out of his or her way to insult that person, then there is a problem. However, if the individual does not act on the feeling of envy and entertains other thoughts or engages in other activities independent of this person, then there is no problem. In fact, this response should be commended. It is not the emotion that is value laden, rather it is the response to that emotion that is value laden.

The Classifications of Emotions

A very common question that arises with the subject of emotions is "Just how many emotions are there?" The question implies a definite answer in terms of numbers. However, the real answer is that there are *countless* emotions. Variability in situations, personal histories, and how people respond gives rise to a high range and number of emotions.

Root emotions. Emotions can be grouped that are variations or nuances of the same root emotion. For example, the emotion of anger can be viewed as a root for the emotions of resentment, hatred, revenge, passive aggression, disgust, hostility, and antagonism. Recovering alcoholics who are struggling with managing their emotions, thoughts, and behaviors, can have the situations simplified, to some extent, by pinpointing the root emotions that may be presently operating in their lives.

The overall approach taken in this book is to classify emotions in terms of the responses or behaviors that *follow* the emotions: a. Potentially constructive, and b. Potentially destructive.

Potentially constructive. These emotions, often called positive emotions, are defined by the positive, encouraging, helpful responses that may follow the emotion. For example, individuals who are feeling the emotion of happiness are likely to say something pleasant and upbeat to other people. Potentially constructive emotions include joy, positive self-esteem, compassion, curiosity, empathy, interest, and passion. The goal of the strategies presented later in this chapter is to increase the occurrences and regularity of these emotions.

Potentially destructive. By contrast, these emotions, often called negative emotions, are defined by the negative, harmful, and unhelpful responses that may follow the emotion. For example, individuals who are feeling the emotion of resentment are likely to act negatively toward some people by insulting them or doing something to cause them harm or embarrassment. Potentially destructive emotions include anger, apathy, fear, shame, resentment, grief, boredom, and low self-esteem.

Emotions as Cyclical

In the following sections, information is provided on this cyclical interplay between the triggers and the components of the environment, emotions, physiological factors, thoughts, behavior and their impact creating an *ongoing cycle.* By understanding this interplay of components as a cycle, recovering alcoholics will be in a stronger position to manage emotions. The approach is to break up the cycle that leads to negative interactions and destructive results, and create a new cycle that leads to positive behavior and constructive results which in this book is called *emotional growth.*

> **Important Perspective**
>
> It cannot be overstated that emotions in themselves are neither good nor bad. Emotions are simply part of our makeup. It is a person's behavior following the emotion that determines the rightness or wrongness of the response for the individual involved.

Managing Emotions

The primary objective in this chapter is to assist recovering alcoholics to manage their emotions. However, emotions themselves are not stand-alone entities that can be directly manipulated. Emotions need to be understood in terms of their interaction between thoughts and behavior. It is the thoughts and behavior that can be manipulated so that in an indirect sense emotions can be managed. For example, a person may have the sensation of strong feelings of fear in a certain situation which could set the occasion for this person to hide or feign sickness to escape. In this case the fear is managed by hiding or feigning sickness. Similarly, a person may feel resentment when she sees someone who reminds her of her abusive ex-husband. She can perseverate on thoughts as to what an evil, no-good, arrogant, and selfish person her ex-husband is (which could lead to aggressive or insulting talk to this person), or she could do her best to push these thoughts aside and focus on something more constructive, such as the things she needs for her garden. In this way the negative thoughts, and possible negative behavior, are prevented.

Cycle of Emotions

Topics for the cycle of emotions include: a. Description of component terms, b. Description of the cycle process, c. Illustrations of the cycle process, and d. Fast-cycle process.

Description of Component Terms

Figure 11.1: Cycle of Emotions depicts a general sequence of events involving six components of emotional behavior. The components in the cycle are: Triggers, Emotions, Physiology, Thinking, Behavior, and Impact. Three components are shaded for identification: Triggers, Thinking, and Behavior. These three shaded components are *targets of intervention* and are controllable. The skills to control them are described later in this section.

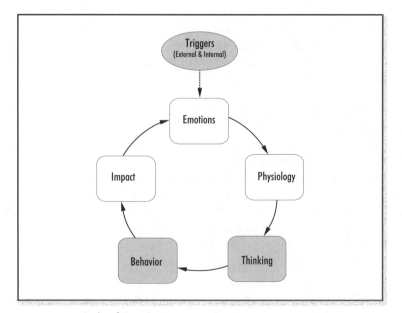

FIGURE 11.1: Cycle of Emotions

Triggers. Anything that sets off emotions is a trigger. Triggers can be controlled as described in the strategies section. Sources of triggers are identified in Figure 11.1 as *External* and *Internal*. External triggers refer to something that happens outside of the individual such as events in the environment with other people or circumstances. For example, the appearance of a friend may elicit the emotion of joy or an altercation at work which can bring about the emotion of anger. Internal triggers refer to thoughts and imaginings that arise in an individual's mind. For example, simply thinking about someone or something can bring forth emotions such a harbored resentment over a certain incident involving another person. The individuals recreate the situation in their mind, identify how they were wronged, and visualize several options for paying this person back, and it is not long before these individuals experience the emotion of revenge.

External events or internal thoughts become emotional triggers because they are associated with some previous history. An event or thought may remind the person of a past situation that caused personal problems or may have been particularly satisfying. For example, someone may make a comment that reminds a person of a similar comment that led to quite a nasty interaction on an earlier occasion. The comment itself, even though it comes in a different context, can trigger emotions because of the association with the previous problematic situation.

Another critical feature regarding triggers is that some individuals can be living in a state of emotions or operating in a certain mood. Consequently, individuals, because of this mood, may interpret an event in a pre-determined manner. For example, if an individual is already feeling angry and someone makes a comment, the comment may be interpreted as offensive or confrontational. Whereas a third person who is relatively calm who heard the comment would say, "Come on now. He meant nothing by that." The implication, as will be noted for recovering alcoholics, is that it is very important to develop strategies for addressing emotional states and moods so that such misperceptions will be minimized.

Emotions. The triggers, by definition, set off or arouse emotions. For the purpose of this book the emotions have been grouped into potentially constructive or potentially destructive. For example, running into a good friend at the mall triggers the emotion of delight in a person. The person smiles and gives the friend a hug. Or, a person is bumped when standing in line at the mall which brings about the emotion of annoyance. Essentially, emotions typically arise in an automatic manner. The position taken in this book is that emotions arise spontaneously or automatically. We cannot directly control whether or not emotions arise. The control lies in what occurs following the arousal of emotions and what happens regarding the triggers.

Physiology. Some emotions can result in bodily changes or physiological reactions. For example, a person feels pain in the chest and thinks it could be heart problems. The person then feels anxious and fearful which results in the person perspiring and trembling. Another person may be watching a sunset and feel an emotion of peace which is accompanied by a physical response of slower breathing and muscle relaxation. The reactions are automatic and are part of the individual's makeup. As with emotions, the position taken in this book is that individuals cannot directly control these physiological reactions. The locus of control is in what happens following the arousal of emotions and physiological reactions and what happens regarding the triggers. Both emotions and physiological reactions are simply viewed as an intrinsic part of an individual's makeup.

Thinking. Once an emotion is present, many thoughts can come to mind for the person. For example, if a person feels the emotions of resentment and revenge, then thoughts of what can be done, how the other person or persons can be made to suffer, and why they deserve to suffer come to mind. In addition, all sorts of thoughts of self-pity and being a victim can arise during this thinking phase which further adds to the intensity of the moment. Thoughts play a critical role in the cycle of emotions. Thoughts can significantly influence the behavioral responses an individual may make following the experience of emotions. Thoughts are one of the major areas where emotions can be managed which will be described more fully in the sections on strategies and steps later in this chapter.

Behavior. The combination of emotions and thoughts often set the occasion for a behavioral response. For example, a person feels angry over a workmate's treatment and begins to think that this workmate deserves some kind of payback. So the person berates the workmate in front of other staff. Or, a person feels grateful for a friend's support and buys a small gift to express the gratitude. Understanding interplay of behaviors with emotions is critical for managing emotions. Controlling one's behavior is central to managing the cycle of emotions. The goal is to develop strategies for building constructive responses to emotions and to reduce destructive responses. Details for this approach will be provided later on in this chapter.

Impact. The action taken by the person following the arousal of emotions and thoughts can have a positive or negative impact on oneself and on others. The result can be constructive or destructive. For example, the person who berated the workmate in front of staff is more than likely to maintain or increase hostilities between the particular workmate (and may have lost some respect from observing staff). This impact was negative or destructive. On the other hand, the person who gave a friend a small gift in gratitude for support is likely to have pleased the friend and strengthened their friendship. Here the impact was positive or constructive.

Maintaining the cycle. The ongoing effect of positive and negative responses to emotions and thoughts is to strengthen the whole cycle. This means that a cycle is established that forms habits. For example, the person who exhibits destructive behaviors following anger, and thoughts associated with anger, is likely to exhibit the same or similar destructive behaviors for future events that triggered the anger. Or, the person who exhibits constructive behaviors following the emotion of gratitude, and thoughts related to gratitude, is likely to show similar behavior in future occasions where gratitude arises.

Description of the Cycle Process

In Figure 11.1: Cycle of Emotions a sequence of stages is presented to describe the process depicting the interplay of the various components for behaviors that are often labeled as an emotional response to a certain situation. The process typically follows this sequence:

1. **Triggers.** It begins with some event or events (internal—thoughts, imaginings; or external—others, events in the environment) that set off emotions.

2. **Emotions.** The triggers arouse emotions (feelings and moods).

3.   **Physiological reaction.** These emotions often cause physiological reactions in one's body.

4.   **Thinking.** Once the person's emotions and physiology have been aroused, thoughts begin to emerge. The thoughts usually center on interpretations of the situation and the possibilities for dealing with it.

5.   **Behavior.** Following some thinking time, which can vary in length, the individual then takes some action or provides a behavioral response.

6.   **Impact.** The actual response has an impact on the situation that can be positive/constructive or it can be negative/destructive. The impact can be directed to self or others.

7.   **Cycle.** The immediate effect of the behavior may be to reduce the emotions or increase them depending on subsequent interactions. The long-term effect will be to strengthen the whole cycle represented by the arrows connecting the components. This means that the individual is likely to make the same constructive or destructive responses in future similar situations.

Illustrations of the Cycle Process

Illustration 1

Sarah is at a birthday gathering for her workmates and is talking with a friend. She looks across the room and sees a woman who is dating her ex-boyfriend. Sarah's ex-boyfriend was quite abusive to her toward the end of their relationship. Seeing this woman at the party was quite a shock *(trigger)*. Sarah felt resentment rising in her and strong feelings of anger toward this woman and her ex-boyfriend *(emotions)*. She then experienced goose bumps and began to tremble a little *(physiology)*. She thinks that this person must be a real loser to see anything in her ex-boyfirend. She wonders what he is up to and how he might be abusing this new girlfriend. She thinks about saying something to her about whether she knows what a jerk he is. She thinks her ex should never be allowed near another woman and wonders how she might make him pay for the abuse and suffering he caused her *(thinking)*. As it turns out, this woman heads toward Sarah and smiles as she passes. Sarah is further annoyed and sees the smile as a kind of smirk of arrogance *(additional trigger)*. Sarah becomes quite annoyed and says, "So how's that dumb … *(expletive)*? Tell him my life is wonderful now that he has dragged himself off to you" *(behavior)* The woman pauses, then whispers, "I see why he ditched you," and moves away very quickly *(negative impact)*.

Comments

1. In this example the presence of the woman who is currently dating Sarah's abusive ex-boyfriend became a strong reminder of the bad experience Sarah had with her ex-boyfriend. The anger she holds for her ex becomes associated with Sarah.

2. The thoughts Sarah has are laced with anger and her need to punish or pay back her ex for what he has done to her.

3. Sarah reads the woman's smile as a smirk—a negative interpretation because she is so angry and can see no good in her ex or anyone associated with him.

4. Sarah's response to the woman is negative and destructive resulting in a cutting reply from the woman. The overall impact is that Sarah's anger toward her ex has been further hardened and now she will bear a grudge against this woman because of her hurtful response. This cycle will continue.

Illustration 2

Renaldo is a 35-year-old recovering alcoholic who has been sober for four years. He has rarely dated during his four years of sobriety. A birthday party was held for one of his co-workers at a local pizza restaurant. Here he is next to a woman he likes. He is very worried about what to say and concerned that she may not like him. He noticed that she was not saying that much either. One of the group mentioned that there was a baseball game on the next day that looked quite exciting and that a couple of them were going. "Anyone else interested?" the coworker asked *(trigger)*. Renaldo asked Elise if she had any interest in baseball *(behavior)* as he held his breath and shook a little through nervousness and a little fear *(physiology)*. She said that she is not a real big fan. Renaldo started to think on whether he should ask her to go with him and the others. A million thoughts seemed to go through his mind, "What if she said no?" "What if she didn't like baseball really?" "Will she think I am putting the make on her as we barely know each other outside of work?" *(thinking)*. As these thoughts went through his mind he felt fearful *(emotions)* and could feel his palms sweating *(physiology)*. He then realized she was looking at him. He kind of blurted out that he is going to the game and wondered if she might like to come along with them *(behavior)*. She smiled and said, "Sure. Sounds like fun." Renaldo felt a huge reduction in tension and was just delighted *(positive impact)*.

Comments

1. This example highlights the difficulties recovering alcoholics face when it comes to social competencies in conversing and becoming more acquainted with another person (discussed in Chapter 10 on the subject of Social Growth).

2. The example also illustrates that the interplay between triggers, emotions, thinking, and behaviors can occur very quickly in an ongoing back-and-forth manner.

3. Renaldo, from his perspective, took a huge leap or risk in asking Elise to go to the game even though it was a relatively safe outing with a group.

4. The pleasing outcome of Elise agreeing to go with him to the game was a very significant positive and constructive result for Renaldo. He experienced relief and delight as a result. He was not only pleased with himself for taking the risk but gratified that she had accepted his offer. He will now have a little more confidence in himself which will carry over to future situations and his relationship with Elise has been strengthened.

Fast-Cycle Process

The concept of a fast cycle is typically used when steps from the normal cycle are omitted for efficiency and economical reasons. For example, dishwashers and washing machines have fast cycles because the load may be small or restricted items are being cleansed. Similarly, in work production situations, a fast cycle may be used to accelerate the completion of a job. There are two common significant applications of this fast cycle concept to the cycle of emotions: a. Omitting the *thinking* phase, and b. Repressing the emotions phase.

Omitting the Thinking Phase

This is very common and is especially important in examining the cycle of emotions. Simply put, many individuals react when emotions arise without thinking about how to respond. For example, when anger is triggered the person reacts immediately by shouting or hitting. Another person may experience great joy over something and act impulsively by walking off their job to celebrate. In other words the thinking phase is passed over. When the thinking phase is omitted, the subsequent behavior is often called impulsive, reactive, self-gratifying, or impetuous.

Young children typically respond to emotions by acting immediately. They do not think about what to do. They just act. It is part of the developmental process for them to learn to process situations, think things through, and act accordingly. It is a sign of maturity to stop and think before acting in demanding or contentious situations. Many adults and particularly recovering alcoholics have not become proficient in using the thinking phase. They simply operate on a fast cycle in going from emotions to behaviors. However, the *thinking* phase and controlling thoughts can be learned and will be addressed in the strategies and steps section later in this chapter.

Repressing the Emotions Phase

This is another way that the normal cycle of emotions can be circumvented. In this fast cycle, an individual passes over the *emotions* phase by repressing or bottling up emotions. For example, a situation may trigger anger and the person just freezes, not allowing the anger to be shown. Another person may be experiencing a death in the family and does not want to communicate any sign of grief. So the person bottles up the grief and tries to tough out the situation. Or, a person may have achieved a significant accomplishment and everyone else wants to celebrate and express their joy, but this person will not accept their accolades and just exhibits a neutral or nonresponsive posture to the attempts of others to reach him or her.

In these examples of fast cycle the individuals have emotions triggered, but they are held in check or not allowed to operate. Consequently, the individual's cycle goes from triggers to thinking to behavior. The emotional phase is omitted (along with the repressed physiological phase).

Repressing emotions is a common strategy for some people to manage their emotions. Basically, they manage their emotions by trying to deny or eliminate them. However, there are several harmful, long-term negative effects that arise for individuals who repress emotions as a standard practice. These negative effects include depression and other mental issues, alcoholism and other addictions, stilted relationships, problems with communication, nurturing difficulties with children, and inability to develop quality of life factors (Billig, 1999; Nelson, 2007).

This particular form of fast cycle for the cycle of emotions is particularly important for recovering alcoholics to understand. One of the most significant effects of alcoholism is that the continued consumption of alcohol serves to repress emotions. Basically, the alcoholic uses alcohol to deal with problem situations. Consequently, the emotions that typically arise for others in these situations are masked or repressed through the alcohol use and abuse. More detail will be provided on this topic in the next section and in the section on general strategies for managing emotions.

The Impact of Alcoholism on Emotions

There is no question that alcoholism has had very serious and harmful effects on emotional states and mood swings for recovering alcoholics. In addition, recovering alcoholics face daunting challenges in their efforts to manage their emotions. This impact of alcoholism on emotions must be examined, understood, and addressed for effective support plans to be developed. Specific topics in this section include: a. Research, b. Emotional needs and alcohol use, c. Agenda for recovering alcoholics, and d. Approach for addressing emotional problems.

Research

Neurobiological damage as a result of alcoholism has been described in Chapter 1 and the systemic effects of impairments to autonomy, cognitive, and social functioning have been addressed in Chapters 8, 9, and 10. There is ample research documenting that brain damage from alcoholism causes alcoholics to process emotions differently from nonalcoholics. Specifically, alcoholics typically misinterpret facial cues of others and have difficulty interpreting nonverbal emotional cues, particularly facial expressions. This means that alcoholics often have flat or nonreceptive responses to people where nonalcoholics would show visible concern or strong responses. In addition, alcoholics show aggression, social inhibition, and impulsivity in certain situations where nonalcoholics display nonreactive behavior, social appropriateness, and control (Fernandez-Serrano, Lozano, Perez-Garcia, & Verdejo-Garcia, 2010; McCoy, 2007; Townsend & Duka, 2003).

Emotional Needs and Alcohol Use

It was noted in Chapter 2 that some individuals turn to alcohol as a way of dealing with strong emotions. For example, individuals may be fearful in the presence of others because they are inhibited when it comes to talking to people. However, after they have had a few drinks they discover they become relaxed, are able to communicate, and the fear disappears. Other individuals may have significant worries about work or family and also find that alcohol can significantly lessen these worries. Alcohol serves them by reducing emotional stress.

Another common reason people turn to alcohol is to enhance emotions. Some individuals are feeling pleased because of some successful situation or an event arises that needs to be recognized. So they turn to alcohol to celebrate. Alcohol has the effect of making the group or individuals feel happier, more relaxed, and joyful.

In each of these situations, alcohol served to alter the individuals' emotions. In the first case, negative emotions (fear and worry) were reduced or removed. In the second situation, positive emotions were enhanced. Some individuals may turn to alcohol more frequently to experience these results and become alcoholics (see Chapter 2). The management of emotions plays a critical role in establishing alcoholism and in establishing a healthy and sober lifestyle.

Agenda for Recovering Alcoholics

Recovering alcoholics have made a most laudable accomplishment in becoming sober. However, they are not out of the woods by a long shot when it comes to managing emotions for three major reasons:

1. Emotional needs were a significant factor why individuals became alcoholics in the first place (such as to reduce anxiety, cope with inhibitions or depression, or the desire for enhancement). Alcohol has simply served to suppress these emotions and once sober these suppressed emotional needs return. For individuals who used alcohol for enhancement, a *void* will emerge. They feel the need to party, celebrate, and have fun, but they are left without a way to fulfill this need. So when they go to an event and do not drink, they feel flat.

In each case, the re-emergence of suppressed emotions or the impact of a void typically causes havoc in the emotional life of the recovering alcoholic. The dry drunk syndrome, described in Chapter 7, captures the confusion, frustration, disappointment, and social ineptness that recovering alcoholics often experience, especially early in sobriety.

2.   The drinking and drunk period of alcoholism puts individuals in a zone where they rarely have the need to respond to their own emotions, respond to others, or deal with problems. Many skills are put on hold when they are drinking heavily. However, when they become sober a stark reality sets in that they have skill deficits in a multitude of situations, be it communicating with others, managing their own affairs, or dealing with issues. They are then very likely to become anxious and stressed out over their ineptness. This situation can become very troublesome because on the one hand they feel positive in that they are sober, and yet the reality of living day to day becomes emotionally distressing.

3.   It has been reported in research, noted in an earlier section of this chapter, that alcoholics' perception of emotional needs or moods of others is distorted compared to nonalcoholics. This finding has serious implications for the emotional and social growth for recovering alcoholics. For example, a person may be quite upset and is looking sad and distressed. The recovering alcoholic may perceive that this person is thinking and nonchalantly ask, "So what's on your mind?" The person, however, is put off by this remark as insensitive and inappropriately prying. The implication is that the recovering alcoholic, because of the harmful effects of sustained use of alcohol, has to develop a new set of skills in understanding and recognizing emotional signs in others and themselves.

Approach for Addressing Emotional Problems

Once recovering alcoholics become sober, they face a number of challenges in key areas of autonomous, cognitive, social, and emotional growth. The approach taken in this book is that these problems have their roots in skill deficits and that recovering alcoholics can be taught to become reasonably proficient in these skill areas. The primary intervention in this chapter, as in previous Chapters 8, 9, and 10, is to describe strategies to teach recovering alcoholics how to manage their emotional needs. These general strategies and specific steps, are described in the next two sections.

General Strategies for Managing Emotions

There is a very important premise in this section. An individual's emotions *can be managed*. While the makeup of emotions varies from individual to individual, there are certain effective strategies that can be used to prevent emotions taking control of the individual. The goal is for recovering alcoholics to recognize that an array of emotions may be experienced and take measures to ensure these emotions foster constructive behavior and prevent emotions from precipitating destructive behavior. The overall intent is to work with emotions so that a positive cycle of emotions is established.

There are several general strategies and specific steps that have proven to be helpful for recovering alcoholics, and nonalcoholics for that matter, in managing emotions. General strategies include: a. Understanding the windows for managing emotions, and b. Classifying emotions.

Understanding the Windows for Managing Emotions

In Figure 11.1, Cycle of Emotions, six phases were described (triggers, emotions, physiology, thinking, behavior, and impact). Three of these phases are considered to be automatic (emotions, physiology, and impact). For example, someone pushes in line at the post office. The person whose place is taken feels a burst of annoyance or anger (the emotion of anger is aroused automatically). A woman is waiting in the lobby for an interview and feels quite anxious and notices her palms are slightly sweaty and that she is tapping her feet on the floor (the sweaty palms and feet tapping are automatic physiological reactions to being nervous before her interview). Another individual is resentful over someone else's promotion at work, begins to vent quite loudly about the situation at a gathering, and the group begins to dissolve and move away from the individual (the impact of the individual's outburst in breaking up the group is predictable and automatically linked to the behavior).

The other three phases are the locus for intervention in managing emotions (triggers, thinking, and behavior). For example, when recovering alcoholics can identify the triggers that set off their emotions, they are in a position to directly manipulate these triggers so that the emotions are lessened or changed. Or, when individuals feel strong emotions are present, they can think about them and what to do. Their thinking can focus on the merits of each response and make an informed and constructive choice. Finally, when the person acts or chooses a certain behavior in response to the situation, the impact is more likely to be constructive.

It is by the planned use of strategies designed to manipulate triggers, thinking, and behavior that recovering alcoholics can be more effective in managing their emotions and live a life of healthier sobriety.

Classifying Emotions

One of the most important steps when it comes to addressing emotions and developing strategies is to pinpoint which emotions are operating with an individual, what triggers these emotions and the behavior typically displayed when these emotions are present. This information gives the recovering alcoholic a basis for selecting which strategies to use and can provide an index for measuring progress.

The identification and classification of human emotions has been the subject of research, conceptual analysis, and practice for many years. For example, Plutchik (1980) developed a widely used model known as *Plutchik's Wheel of Emotions*; Ortony and Turner (1990) compiled a list of basic emotions derived from major theorists; and Parrot (2001) developed a conceptual framework showing the relationship between emotions in terms of primary, secondary, and tertiary categorizations.

Recovering alcoholics could easily get lost in this maze of information on emotions. They need a simple way to identify the major emotions that come into play in their lives. The critical question becomes "What are the predominant emotions that arise in the lives of recovering alcoholics?" The approach taken in this book is to carefully examine the widely adopted resource book for recovering alcoholics, *Alcoholics Anonymous* and identify the most frequently cited emotions (including their derivatives and synonyms). *The Big Book Concordance* (Roy Y., 1997), an index for all words appearing in the text of the third edition of *Alcoholics Anonymous,* was used for this search. These findings, in conjunction with the general literature on classifying emotions, are presented in Box 11.1. This list is for recovering alcoholics to identify the prevailing emotions in their lives. The results of this search for positive or potentially constructive emotions and negative or potentially destructive emotions are presented in Box 11.1. The emotions in this list have been distilled from over 1300 to a more manageable number. These emotions are also included as part of this chapter's checklist and action plan (at the end of this chapter, Illustration 11.3, and Appendix P: Form 11.3, Checklist and Action Plan for Developing Emotional Growth).

BOX 11.1: Counts of Positive and Negative Emotions Cited in Alcoholics Anonymous (3rd ed).	
Count	Emotion (Derivatives and Synonyms)
POSITIVE OR POTENTIALLY CONSTRUCTIVE EMOTIONS	
184	1. Joyful: happy excited, exhilarant, jubilant, merry, exalted, cheer, glad, elated, proud
179	2. Loving: love, affection, care, compassion, kind, generous. courageous
112	3. Peaceful: comfortable, serene, mellow, relish, calm, fulfilled, satisfied, modest, humble
95	4. Hopeful: hope, optimism, desiring, wanting, goal directed, needful.
44	5. Grateful: thankful, gratitude, appreciative,
Total: 625	
NEGATIVE OR POTENTIALLY DESTRUCTIVE EMOTIONS	
168	1. Fearful: afraid, frightened, terrified, threatened, insecure
151	2. Angry: hateful, fury, irritable, rage, resentment, antipathy, offended, disgusted, annoyed
111	3. Anxious: dismayed, distressed, perturbed, worried, frustrated, edgy, needful
159	4. Depressed: hopeless, despair, discouraged, disheartened, miserable, morbid, apathy, boredom, sadness, despondent, disappointed.
88	5. Self-Pity: pained, injured, sick, tired, excuses, envy, jealousy, lonliness, alone, rejected
Total: 677	

Source: Big Book Concordance, www.royy.com/concord.html

Specific Steps for Managing Emotions

In Figure 11.1, Cycle of Emotions, six phases were depicted. The strategies for addressing emotional growth, either to increase the effects of positive emotions or to decrease the effects of negative emotions, are focused on *three shaded* phases in the Figure 11.1: Cycle of Emotions—namely triggers, thinking, and behavior.

The other three unshaded phases in the figure (emotions, physiology, and impact), are considered to be automatic dependent factors that cannot be directly manipulated by strategies.

The overall objectives when addressing emotions is to pinpoint which constructive emotions need to be built up and which destructive ones need to be minimized; determine the triggers for these emotions; and develop a comprehensive plan to manage and control the emotions. There are three steps for accomplishing these objectives: 1. Identify the target emotions, 2. Determine the operating triggers for these emotions, and 3. Select strategies for developing positive emotions and reducing the impact of negative emotions. These three steps are then combined to produce a comprehensive checklist and action plan Form 11.3: Comprehensive Checklist and Action Plan for Developing Emotional Growth (Appendix P).

Step 1 Identify the Target Emotions

In this initial step the individual provides background information for classifying emotions then follows a checklist designed to pinpoint which emotions need to be developed and/or curtailed. These selections are then prioritized.

Pinpointing and Prioritizing Emotions

Given that there is a vast array of emotions that can come into play in the daily lives of all people, including recovering alcoholics, it is important to have a way of pinpointing which emotions are of importance for personal growth. The checklist presented in Form 11.1, Appendix N, is drawn from Box 11.1. Major emotions are listed along with their derivatives and synonyms. The recovering alcoholics are encouraged to work through this list choosing *Yes* for emotions important to them at this time. In the second half of the form, the selections are prioritized. One or two of the *No* emotions are selected from the first column and one or two of the *Yes* emotions are selected from the second column (at least one from each group of positive and negative emotions). These prioritized selections will then become the target emotions for determining the triggers (Form 11.2, Appendix O) and in developing a comprehensive intervention plan (Form 11.3, Appendix P). An example of a completed Form 11.1 is presented in Illustration 11.1

Background: Micheil is a 41-year-old with 8 years of sobriety, very active in the Fellowship of AA devoting much of his time to doing service work. In his efforts as a sponsor he lost three sponsees who sought other sponsors. In addition, he was not elected to the last three service positions for which he stood. Micheil, in talking with his sponsor and some friends, received the feedback that he is quite hostile, hard to get on with, and has all the characteristics of a dry drunk. On the other hand, he is very devoted to his family and it gives him great joy to play games with the children and to go on walks with his wife and family. His sponsor encouraged him to work on his emotions and begin by completing the following form. His sponsor knew that Micheil would not complete the form accurately (part of the dry-drunk syndrome) so they agreed to complete it together.

ILLUSTRATION 11.1: Checklist for Determining Target Emotions

Positive Emotions	Selection (Underline)	Negative Emotions	Selection (Underline)
1. Joyful: happy, excited, exhilarant, jubilant, merry, exalted, cheer, glad, elated, proud	<u>Yes</u> No	**1. Fearful:** afraid, frightened, terrified, threatened, insecure	Yes <u>No</u>
2. Loving: love, affection, care, compassion, kind, generous. courageous	<u>Yes</u> No	**2. Angry:** hateful, fury, irritable, rage, resentment, antipathy, offended, disgusted, annoyed	<u>Yes</u> No
3. <u>Peaceful</u>: comfortable, serene, mellow, relish, calm, fulfilled, satisfied, modest, humble	Yes <u>No</u>	**3. <u>Anxious</u>:** dismayed, distressed, perturbed, worried, frustrated, edgy, needful	<u>Yes</u> No
4. Hopeful: hope, optimism, desiring, wanting, goal directed, needful.	Yes <u>No</u>	**4. <u>Depressed</u>:** hopeless, despair, discouraged, disheartened, miserable, morbid, apathy, boredom, sadness, despondent, disappointed	<u>Yes</u> No
5. <u>Grateful</u>: thankful, gratitude, appreciative	Yes <u>No</u>	**5.Self-Pity:** pained, injured, sick, tired, excuses, envy, jealousy, lonliness, alone, rejected	Yes <u>No</u>
Positive Emotions Results Prioritize No Selections (1 or 2 only) 1. *Peaceful* 2. *Grateful*		**Negative Emotions Results** Prioritize Yes Selections (1 or 2 only) 3. *Depressed* 4. *Anxious*	

Step 2 Determine the Operating Triggers

A wide variety of factors can occur in daily life that can impact emotions. For example, a telemarketing phone call during dinner, rejection at work, a surprise gift in the mail, a planned visit from a close friend, dealing with pain and discomfort, a loud noise, a smelly room, a baby's cry or smile, a branch fallen across a fence in the backyard, and sustained insufficiency of funds can trigger the full array of emotions. These events and effects are considered to be typical or normal in life and most people learn to cope with such triggers and manage the effects appropriately.

The recovering alcoholic, however, can be overcome by such triggers and become despondent, experience relapses with drinking, or adopt other inappropriate responses. It is very important in the recovery process, especially in relation to developing personal growth, to identify the external and internal triggers that lead to emotional problems such as becoming angry, fearful, resentful, and envious (or whatever emotions are involved). Once these feelings become present, unless steps are taken, the recovering alcoholic may exhibit behavior that is destructive or counterproductive. A critical step for controlling the impact of negative emotions and for enhancing the effects of positive emotions is to identify the triggers that bring on these emotions in the first place. Once the triggers are identified, strategies can be applied to help manage emotions that may arise. We will describe several common major triggers which may be presently operating in the life of the recovering alcoholic. The descriptions are followed by Illustration 11.2.

Common Major Triggers

1. **Thoughts.** One of the most challenging trigger sources of emotions for recovering alcoholics are thoughts, especially negative thoughts. A person can be sitting having a cup of coffee and then thoughts arise, as if from nowhere, about some past incident or some new development, negative feelings emerge, the mind starts to run and before long strong feelings are generated. The challenge is that thoughts can arise at any time during the day or evening at predictable times and also at unexpected times.

2. **Communication.** There are endless opportunities for triggers to operate under the broad category of communication (such as something that arises from reading the newspaper, book, or magazine, watching TV, having a conversation with friends, a text message on a cell phone, or an email message). We

can be literally inundated with information in many different ways. Not surprisingly, at times this information or communication can set the stage for negative feelings.

3. **Reminders or Flashbacks**. It is not uncommon for a situation to trigger strong emotions because the person is reminded of earlier circumstances that were traumatic, difficult, distressing, and in general quite negative. Here are some examples of these triggers:

    "The way you said that reminded me of my father who was abusive to me when I was a child. I just felt a burst of fear."

    "I stayed at this hotel when I had a big argument with my ex several years back and I have the same hostile feelings again."

    "When you say, 'Drop in and watch the game,' I am reminded of the times I would do that and get drunk. Your invitation makes me nervous."

4. **Unresolved Conflicts**. It is relatively common for people to experience conflicts with others that were not dealt with or resolved. These conflicts can occur within families, between friends, at the work site, or in business arrangements. For example, one person may receive a promotion or favor over another which can lead to ongoing resentment. Two family members may get into a dispute resulting in a stand-off where neither of them talks to the other again. A person may feel short-changed with a job done on their car. Consequently, when these individuals come in contact again negative feelings are likely to arise.

5. **Breakdowns in Relationships**. An individual, family, or group of people, may inflict harm, damage, insult, or unfair treatment of a person. This hurt may be sustained and ill feelings harbored so that subsequent encounters trigger negative emotions. For example, a family member may feel unfairly slighted because he or she was left out of a will or not involved with some decisions the family made. A workmate may be isolated and not invited to attend parties or company events. Subsequent contact with these individuals or group, or others associated with them, can generate negative emotions.

6.   **Adapting to Changes.** Clearly, daily living involves adapting to changes such as a change of plans, re-locating, finding a job, disruption of routines, going through separation or divorce, transitions such as finishing school, starting a business, or having friends or family leave town. Some people cope well with changes while others have trouble making the necessary adaptations and can experience a full array of negative emotions such as anger, panic, confusion, and resentment. By contrast, in other cases, these same changes can trigger constructive emotions such as excitement, hope, enthusiasm, and eagerness to succeed.

7.   **Making Decisions.** The need to make decisions in a timely manner can trigger negative emotions for some people. Problems known as seasonal affective disorders (SAD) are brought on by long periods of dreary, overcast skies. Some individuals may panic, become fearful, or choke when decisions have to be made. The problems can be accentuated when the decisions are tied to other events that are causing problems. For example, a person may have lost his or her job and has to make a decision on how the holiday season will be spent.

8.   **Impact of Environment.** Environmental factors can trigger negative emotions such as relentless climatic conditions (heat, cold, wind, rain, or snow). Similarly, living conditions can also play a role in triggering negative emotions. For example, an apartment complex may be too noisy or unsafe, the roads may be too dusty, offensive odors may persistently come from a nearby paper mill, sewage plant, or refuse site.

9.   **Health Issues.** Health issues often can trigger negative emotions. Persons with chronic pain, temporary disabilities, onset of pain and discomfort. Pain can put people on edge so that negative emotions of anger, frustration, despair, panic, self-pity, and fear can readily surface.

10.   **Marginal Living.** Some recovering alcoholics' living situations are best described as marginal. They could be living off and on the streets or in temporary housing, have insufficient funds for meals, clothing, and other basic needs. These situations can readily trigger destructive emotions of fear, panic, insecurity, and depression.

11. **Victim Dispositions.** Some individuals become alcoholics in the first place because alcohol helps them to deal with, albeit temporarily, being a victim alleviating feelings of self-pity, being misunderstood, being unjustly maligned, and a that's-not-fair mentality. These people will experience the same emotions as recovering alcoholics. The same victim-related emotions will re-emerge once the alcohol intervention is withdrawn.

12. **Social Ineptness.** Similarly, some individuals may turn to drinking and become alcoholics in order to deal with their inhibitions at social events. Consequently, when they become sober, especially initially, they will experience the very same feelings of social ineptness such as shyness, inhibitions, timidity, or inability to communicate.

13. **Personal Issues.** Each person has their own makeup and their own idiosyncrasies. Certain things can trigger emotions with one person and not another. One person may feel strongly about punctuality and lateness can trigger negative emotions. Some people react to things differently. For example, loud talk, body noises, and interruptions can upset some and not others. It is important to identify these unique or personal factors that can serve as triggers for negative emotions.

14. **Personal Safety.** The instinct of personal survival is strong with most people. Consequently, threats to safety can serve as triggers for a full array of emotions such as anger, panic, fear, and anxiety.

15. **Personal Satisfaction.** Recovering alcoholics are often steered toward addressing triggers that lead to negative emotions. It is also important to address, and build upon, those triggers that lead to positive and constructive emotions such as joy, satisfaction, pleasure, and calm.

16. **Other.** Just as there is a vast number of emotions that can come into play in the life of an individual, there is also an extensive list of triggers that may set off these emotions. The fifteen triggers presented in this section are designed to help recovering alcoholics identify the most common triggers in their lives. However, there may be other triggers that come readily to mind once the recovering alcoholic begins the process of identifying these key triggers. It is important for the recovering alcoholic to include these additional

triggers under the item Other in Form 11.2: Checklist for Determining Major Triggers.

Identification of Major Triggers

In Illustration 11.1 the recovering alcoholic (Micheil) identified the major emotions operating in his life. The next step, Form 11.2: Checklist for Determining Operating Triggers (Appendix O), is designed to assist the recovering alcoholics to pinpoint the triggers for their most common emotions. In using Form 11.2, the recovering alcoholic is encouraged to list the prioritized emotions indentified in Form 11.1 and then work through this list of triggers in Form 11.2 choosing *Yes* if a particular item serves as a trigger for the prioritized emotions. The column in the right-hand part of the form headed *Notes* is used for comments or any salient information regarding a particular trigger. In the lower part of the form, the trigger selections are prioritized by selecting two or three triggers that have been scored *Yes*. These results will then be used as a basis for developing a comprehensive intervention plan to address emotions (Form 11.3). An example of a completed Form 11.2 is presented in Illustration 11.2.

Background: Micheil (41 years old, 8 years sober, employed family man) has indicated the following from Illustration 11.1:

    Joyful, *Yes*; Loving, *Yes*; Peaceful, *No*; Hopeful, *No*; Grateful, *No*;

    Fearful, *No*; Angry, *Yes*; Anxious, *Yes*; Depressed, *Yes*; Self-pity, *No*.

He has prioritized four emotions: 1. Peaceful, 2. Grateful; 3. Depressed, 4. Anxious.

Prioritized List of Positive Emotions from Form 11.1	Prioritized List of Negative Emotions from Form 11.1
1. *Peaceful*	3. *Depressed*
2. *Grateful*	4. *Anxious*

ILLUSTRATION 11.2: Checklist for Determining Operating Triggers

Triggers	Selection (Underline) Yes or No	Notes
1. Thoughts	<u>Yes</u> No	*Negative thoughts occur all the time making me resentful.*
2. Communication	<u>Yes</u> No	*I react and get angry when things are said without making much effort to understand what is said.*
3. Reminders or flashbacks	<u>Yes</u> No	*I often am reminded of bad times.*
4. Unresolved conflicts	<u>Yes</u> No	*There are lots of these. Don't know where to start.*

ILLUSTRATION 11.2 *Continued*

5. Breakdown in relationships	Yes <u>No</u>		*I am pretty tight with my family, believe it or not. Brings me joy.*
6. Adapting to changes	Yes <u>No</u>		*I'm okay here I think*
7. Making decisions	Yes <u>No</u>		*Okay here.*
8. Impact of environment	Yes <u>No</u>		*Fine.*
9. Health issues	Yes <u>No</u>		*Okay.*
10. Marginal living	Yes <u>No</u>		*We are okay. My wife has a good job and I can make enough money.*
11. Victim dispositions	<u>Yes</u> No		*Okay.*
12. Social ineptness	<u>Yes</u> No		*Yes, I feel things are stacked against me a lot.*
13. Personal issues	<u>Yes</u> No		*I struggle here with meeting friends, going out with others, having people over, and keeping sponsees.*
14. Personal safety	Yes <u>No</u>		*Okay here.*
15. Other	Yes <u>No</u>		*I'm sure there are, but I have enough already I am fully aware of.*

RESULTS: Prioritize Yes Selections (2 or 3) Operating Triggers

1. *Thoughts*
2. *Communication*
3. *Unresolved conflicts*

Step 3 Select Strategies for Developing Positive Emotions and Reducing Negative Emotions

There is a wide range of strategies for recovering alcoholics to use in addressing their emotional growth. These strategies have been organized around the following sections: a. Maintaining selected initial strategies for achieving sobriety; b. Utilizing strategies for developing *autonomous, cognitive,* and *social* growth; c. Managing the triggers; d. Managing thoughts in the thinking and trigger phases; and e. Establishing replacement behaviors.

Maintaining Selected Initial Strategies for Achieving Sobriety

Even though the focus of this chapter is on expanding recovering alcoholics' skills to address emotional growth, some of the strategies recovering alcoholics used to achieve sobriety in the first place may need to be maintained. For some, these practices are necessary to maintaining sobriety in the long haul and for that reason are considered to be lifelong habits. The situation is analogous to an individual who was very much overweight. The person undertook a weight-loss program and was successful in losing a considerable amount of weight. Once the weight had been lost, the individual still had to maintain certain practices in order to keep the weight down as well as introduce other healthy practices that were not utilized when the person was overweight.

The most common and most effective practices recovering alcoholics use in the early stages of sobriety have been described in earlier chapters, including the following:

- Attend meetings

- Work with a sponsor or support person

- Keep a log or journal

- Use active reflection

- Develop new routines to replace previous drinking places and practices

- Take steps to develop fellowship or new social networks

The recovering alcoholic will know which of these practices should be kept and which should always be resurrected if needed.

Utilizing Strategies for Developing Autonomous, Cognitive, and Social Growth

It was no accident that *emotional* growth is targeted as the fourth key area for recovering alcoholics. It is assumed that growth in other areas, *autonomous, cognitive,* and *social*, needs to be addressed *before* emotional growth is targeted. Growth in these three key areas is considered to be a *protective factor* when it comes to helping a recovering alcoholic control the effects of emotions. Protective factors are those practices that prevent or minimize the vulnerability of a person, in this case—in managing emotions.

Autonomous Skills. If recovering alcoholics take steps to successfully assume more responsibility for their lives, Chapter 8, then they will become more confident and effects of the emotion of *fearful* will be reduced and the effects of the emotion *joyful* or *peaceful* will be increased.

Cognitive Skills. Similarly, if the recovering alcoholic learns to be more effective with problem solving, a strategy described for cognitive growth (Chapter 9), then there are likely to be fewer situations that foster angry and frustrated emotions, and more situations fostering joyful, peaceful, fulfilled, and hopeful emotions.

Social Skills. If the recovering alcoholic learns to develop better skills in the area of social growth (Chapter 10), then the individual will have more success socially and not experience to the same extent the emotion of loneliness.

Recovering alcoholics are strongly encouraged to review the strategies described in Chapters 8, 9, and 10, in particular the specific checklists and action plans for managing autonomous, cognitive, and social growth. Adoption or extension of these practices may be effective in enhancing the effects of positive emotions (left column of Form 11.1, Appendix N) and reducing the effects of negative emotions (right column of Form 11.1).

Managing the Triggers

Once the triggers have been identified (Form 11.2), strategies can be taken to manage these triggers. This management falls into one of two types: a. Controlling triggers for negative emotions, and b. Enhancing triggers for positive emotions.

Controlling Triggers for Negative Emotions

Once recovering alcoholics identify the triggers giving rise to negative emotions, they are in a position to either *change* those triggers or learn to *cope* with them if change is not possible or desirable. As shown in Figure 11.1: Cycle of Emotions, triggers can be extrinsic (coming from events or other people) or intrinsic (coming from internal thoughts and imaginings).

Addressing Sustained Triggers for Negative Emotions

The basic approach for addressing the triggers that set off negative emotions involves eights steps which are described in detail in Chapter 8 (see p. 133, Solve Problems Effectively, and Form 8.2: Procedural Steps for Solving Problems Effectively). These steps can readily be modified for addressing the triggers for negative emotions. The procedures are designed for more situational and recurring triggers—*sustained triggers*. For example, an individual may get angry because the neighbor plays loud music at night or has a barking dog. Another person may experience fear at work because a coworker is threatening or makes untoward comments. Or, an individual may feel strong resentment because a relative misinterpreted some remarks and will not speak to the individual anymore and spreads negative comments to other relatives. In each of these cases there is a problem that is unsolved that produces negative emotions. The problems need to be addressed and solved through some kind of problem-solving strategy (such as the procedures described in Chapter 8 or work through the problem with a sponsor or support person). If the problem is not addressed, then the negative feelings will persist and the recovering alcoholic's emotional and mental health will be impaired.

Here are key points in a problem-solving plan for addressing these triggers:

- Identify the triggers (cause of the problems)

- List possible options for solving the situation

- Select and implement one or more of the options

- Monitor progress

Coping with Sustained Triggers for Negative Emotions

Sometimes the situation or events that trigger negative emotions cannot be changed—the problem-solving approaches are not effective. For example, regarding the illustrations above, the individual is unable to get the music turned down by a resident in a neighboring apartment; the coworkers have not been responsive to appeals to stop the inappropriate comments and threats and their actions have been too subtle to warrant action by the supervisor; and the relative who will not communicate and is spreading negative comments is intractable. In other words, the recovering alcoholic is stuck with the situation. At this juncture the recovering alcoholic can take some consolation in that the problems were addressed, albeit unsuccessfully, and the next step is to employ *coping skills.* Again, strategies for developing coping skills were addressed in Chapter 8, Form 8.4: Checklist and Action Plan for Coping Skills. Here are summary points for developing coping skills:

- Accept the situation as knowing that it has to be lived with

- Develop routines outside of the problem situation that bring relaxation and pleasure

- Maintain contact with a friend, sponsor, or support person

Addressing On-the-Spot Triggers for Negative Emotions

These triggers refer to those events, situations, and thoughts that happen instantaneously or on-the-spot. For example, a person may cut off an individual in traffic and make the individual angry. Or, the supervisor might enter the room and start reprimanding the worker closest to the door. Another individual, further along in the room, may become anxious and fearful about being next to get a reprimand. Similarly, an individual may be harboring some resentment toward another person and one day, through a chance meeting, this person makes what it perceived as a snide remark. The remark can bring about emotions of anger or jealousy.

The basic approach for managing these on-the-spot triggers is to *refocus or shift attention* to something else. If something sets off emotions with a recovering alcoholic, then it is critical to not let the emotions take hold, fester, or lead to inappropriate action. The recovering alcoholic needs to engage in something else, think of something else, or occupy the mind in constructive ways that lead to productive actions. For example, if someone makes a seemingly provocative or slightly offensive remark to an individual triggering a rush of annoyance, then the individual may ignore the remark, talk to someone else, look out the window and check the weather, get busy with some activity, and basically move on from the person making the remark.

Enhancing Triggers for Positive Emotions

A recovering alcoholic asked this insightful question: "Why is it so easy to have negative emotions like getting angry and it is so hard to get positive emotions like being peaceful?" This comment gets to the heart of dealing with emotions. It is analogous to the person who says, "Why is it so easy to gain weight and so difficult to lose it?"

The challenge facing recovering alcoholics when it comes to using practices to develop positive emotions like joy, peace, pleasure, serenity, and happiness is that *new habits* need to be established. Developing positive emotions were not a priority for alcoholics when they were drinking. In fact, alcoholic individuals developed a lot of bad habits that were counterproductive for developing positive emotions. The effects of alcohol masked these issues or rather buried them. However, the recovering alcoholic can take concrete steps to turn this situation around. There is hope.

The steps for enhancing positive emotions are quite systematic and summarized as follows:

- Understand that success will take time and that the recovering alcoholic must be persistent and patient.

- Identify activities that bring enjoyment, peace, and other positive emotions, such as: taking regular walks, working out at the gym, gardening, listening to music or playing an instrument, reading, hobbies, and taking classes (see Chapter 8).

- Develop a routine so that some of these practices are scheduled on a daily or regular basis.

- Establish or join a circle of friends who enjoy similar activities.

- Actively reflect on the effects of these activities for enhancing positive emotions.

Basically, the assumption is that if recovering alcoholics adopt practices that are likely to generate positive emotions, these very activities will become *triggers* for these emotions which, in turn, lead to a higher quality of life.

Managing Thoughts in the Thinking and Trigger Phases

The cyclical relationship between thoughts, emotions, and behavior has been well documented and extensively explored in published treatment and therapy literature (Beck, 1995; Contreras, 2010; Gallagher, 1993). We are all familiar with this relationship in practice. Here are two examples often perceived as internal triggers: a. we only have to think about a serious event in our past for several seconds and it is not long before feelings arise about that event, and b. if we think about a very positive situation for a while, positive emotions begin to arise.

The thinking phase which follows the triggers, emotions, and physiology phases (see Figure 11.1, p. 211) is just what the name implies. It is the time to think and manage thoughts. It is time to stop and think. If we are presently in a situation that has constantly caused us problems and we dwell on the injustices, miscommunications, and harm caused, we are likely to react to the situation and do something we may regret. Management of thoughts is crucial for setting the stage of positive emotions and for leading to constructive behavior. Conversely, if the thoughts are not managed properly then negative emotions may arise followed by destructive behavior. Thoughts play a decidedly critical role in managing emotions and behavior. As the great Roman emperor Marcus Aurelius so aptly said many centuries ago: "The universe is change; our life is what our thoughts make it."

Recovering alcoholics have an additional challenge in managing thoughts. In their drinking days alcohol served to *suppress* unwelcome thoughts and emotions, over many years in some cases. So when these individuals become sober, there is an eruption of thoughts and emotions causing considerable turmoil. Quality recovery programs provide adequate support for alcoholics during this critical initial stage of sobriety. However, once the person has stabilized to some extent, there is a real need to develop strategies to systematically manage thoughts as a key to ongoing emotional growth. The classic *dry drunk* is the epitome of a recovering alcoholic who has not learned to manage thoughts and emotions. These needy people continue to suppress their thoughts and emotions, much as they did when they were drinking, and display behavior similar to when they were drinking. Suppressing thoughts is not a healthy way to manage thoughts.

Reducing Destructive Thoughts and Increasing Constructive Ones

Two broad areas need to be addressed in managing thoughts. First, reducing thoughts that lead to negative emotions and destructive behavior and, second, increasing thoughts that lead to positive emotions and constructive behavior.

These strategies are intended to assist recovering alcoholics in managing negative thoughts when they arise, preventing negative thoughts from occurring in the first place, and encouraging positive thoughts. Note: These procedures are not designed to *suppress* the thoughts. Rather the intent is to *manage or defuse* them.

- **Understand that thoughts can be controlled**. An individual does not have to be enslaved by thoughts. Thoughts can be changed.

- **Understand that thoughts are not facts.** Individuals who worry, for example, must not take their thoughts as the true situation. An elderly person once remarked "I have lived a full life with many crises, most of which never happened." Individuals need to explore what is going on and have a set line when the negative thoughts arise, such as "I will look into this" or "I will check the evidence." Sometimes it is helpful to search for alternative explanations that are not threatening.

- **Understand that negative thoughts are normal or common.** Just because a recovering alcoholic may be consumed by negative thoughts, it does not mean the person is sick, deranged, or abnormal. Being consumed by negative thoughts is a common human phenomenon.

- **Focus on action**. Avoid words like "should," "could," and "ought to." Use words like "will." For example, "At 5 pm today I will go for a walk." These action words help to generate confidence and belief in self which is crucial for managing emotions. Some individuals may become so swamped in emotions, such as those who become seriously depressed, that they become powerless. It is most important for them to focus on action. The catch phrase "Do it anyway" can be helpful. Similarly, a common tool used with AA members is to "Fake it till you make it." Sometimes recovering alcoholics and their sponsors have developed a grid, such as a 3 x 3 table in which up to nine common tasks are written. The recovering alcoholic selects some of these tasks, maybe three, and fulfils them. Over time all tasks are completed—some of these on a daily basis. Other tasks, once completed, are replaced by new challenges.

- **Utilize calming procedures.** Certain activities can help to put a person's mind at rest, such as going for a walk, listening to some relaxing music, and using breathing relaxation exercises. As the individual calms down or becomes more settled, it is easier to shift the mind's focus to more positive thoughts. Meditation, which is described more fully later in this section, is an excellent calming activity.

- **Use a journal**. For some recovering alcoholics, it is helpful to write down their feelings as they occur, write down what it is that is triggering them, and review what is written at a later date. Often, at a later time the individual will conclude that the triggers were not that significant and really did not warrant such a reaction. Individuals may joke with themselves, saying, "You mean I got upset over this? I need to get a life!" In other cases, however, the information may be more serious, especially if it recurs in their thoughts and emotions, and warrants action. Then the individual may need to problem solve or take the issue up with a friend, sponsor, or professional therapist.

- **Contact support**. Recovering alcoholics have been encouraged to contact a friend, support person, or sponsor when tough problems arise. It can be very helpful for an individual who is struggling with negative thoughts and subsequent emotions to call, text, email, or visit with a support person. Simply talking or texting it through can be very helpful.

- **Change the focus**. Thoughts have to have a focus. Negative thoughts focus on a person or persons, events, or circumstances. An effective strategy is to think of something else, change activities, read something, do something else. Essentially, the mind cannot think of two things at the same time. So the recovering alcoholic, when beleaguered with a negative thought or thoughts, must shift the focus to other thoughts or activities. Simply engage the mind in something else, preferably something positive and uplifting but something engaging.

- **Focus on something positive**. Recall an event that made you laugh or happy. Visualize the setting and focus on details in the setting. Some recovering alcoholics have noted improvement in managing negative emotions by developing a sense of gratitude by reflecting on the good things in their lives, things they can be grateful for, especially any positive things that have happened recently.

- **Use tokens and reminders**. One common strategy for changing thought patterns is to carry a token, some little symbol as a reminder of positive thoughts. One recovering alcoholic carries a photo of his daughter on a key chain which he pulls out when he is bothered by feelings of anxiety. The photo helps to bring some joy to the situation as he looks at the picture of his daughter and is reminded that she needs him.

- **Seeking out positive people.** Sometimes it helps to hang out as much as possible with people who are upbeat, have goals, enjoy life, and can see the bright side of things. By contrast, if the recovering alcoholic, who may be struggling with emotional issues such as depression, anxiety, fear, or anger, hangs out mostly with people who are also down with emotional problems, the situation usually worsens or at least remains the same. The thoughts, attitudes, and behavior of positive people often rub off to other people and help them deal with negative emotions.

- **Face the bottom line.** Some individuals who worry, become anxious, and panic about what may happen to them can gain strength by asking these two questions: "What is the worst thing that can happen to me?" followed by "Can I handle it?" Typically, the individuals will conclude that if push comes to shove, they will be able to handle it which, of course, helps to neutralize the negative thoughts.

- **Beware of self-pity and blaming others.** One counterproductive strategy for addressing negative thoughts is to fall into the cycle of self-pity and blaming others. This practice may give some kind of relief but is not helpful in the long run and may lead to a relapse with drinking (discussed in Chapter 12). It is important to try to be objective, look at the triggers, and address the problems, with help as needed.

Adopting a Meditation Practice

Perhaps the least used, least understood, and most effective strategy for managing thoughts and emotions is to practice some form of meditation. Meditation has many approaches and many names such as contemplation, discernment, relaxation exercises, transcendence, centering prayer, and sitting. Recovering alcoholics are encouraged to conduct their own reading and research (much has been written on the subject of meditation), talk to others who meditate regularly, and, above all—try it. In general, the practice of meditation over time enables recovering alcoholics to relax and learn how to deal with their thoughts and emotions.

Here are some common practices used in meditation:

- Schedule a set time and duration for the meditation (for example, after shower in the morning for 20 minutes).

- Designate a quiet spot in the home for the meditation. Some individuals make a small shrine in their home to symbolize the practice.

- Join a group that meditates regularly.

- Select a meditation posture that is comfortable but not likely to have you fall asleep: sitting, kneeling, and using forms of yoga postures and various forms of benches for sitting or kneeling.

- Use breathing exercises to quieten the body and mind.

- Focus the head and the mind.

- Use strategies for managing thoughts, images, distractions, and day-dreaming such as breathing exercises and letting the thoughts come and go or return to a key thought or prayer to provide a focus.

Meditation practice effectively manages thoughts fosters emotional growth, and it has many other benefits. The various forms of meditation are loosely grouped into three approaches: relaxing the mind and body; exercising the mind, and journeying inward. Steps are suggested for using these approaches to meditation and individual recovering alcoholics are encouraged to check out the various approaches and, most importantly, make a start and develop a practice that best suits their own needs.

Additional resources for learning how to meditate are listed in Box 11.2:

BOX 11.2: Additional Resources for the Practice of Meditation

Boud, D., Keogh, R., & Walker, D. (1985). *Reflection: Turning Experience into Learning.* New York: Routledge.

Geoff C., & Scott W. (2011). The Challenge of the 11th Step: Sustaining the Practice of Meditation: Part I, Why Meditate? Emerald Valley Intergroup Newsletter, April, pp. 1, 3, 7.

Geoff C., & Scott W. (2011). The Challenge of the 11th Step: Sustaining the Practice of Meditation: Part II, Some Guidelines for Meditation. *Emerald Valley Intergroup Newsletter,* July, pp. 1, 5.

Davis, M., Robbins, E., McKay, M., & Fanning, P. (2008). *The Relaxation & Stress Reduction Workbook (New-Harbinger Self-Help Workbook).* Oakland, CA: New Harbinger Publications.

Michie, D. (2008). *Hurry Up and Meditate: Your Starter Kit for Inner Peace and Better Health.* Crows Nest, Australia: Allen & Unwin.

Establishing Replacement Behaviors

At this juncture two of the three main areas for using strategies to addressing emotions have been described, *triggers* and *thoughts*. The third major variable is managing *behavior*. The role of behavior is central to managing emotions. For example, one individual experiences the emotion of anger and kicks a hole in the wall of the living room. Another person feels anger and goes for a walk to cool down. Each individual experiences anger, but the subsequent behaviors are markedly different in that one is destructive (kicking a hole in the wall) and the other is constructive (going for a walk). In addition, a crucial question becomes: "What is the individual likely to do the next time anger occurs?" The person who kicked a hole in the wall may become more violent and attack someone or feel guilt over the damage and loss of respect that may result, compounding the emotional impact. By contrast, the person who went for a walk probably experienced some relief as the anger subsided and the next time around would do something similar to cool down when angers arises.

In each of these cases, the individuals experienced the emotion of anger, but the ensuing behavior was different. The key in managing emotions is to use strategies to ensure that constructive behavior follows an emotion and not destructive behavior.

The strategies for managing behavior following negative emotions fall into three areas, or combinations of three areas: first, to delay responding; second, to moderate the emotions; and third, to build constructive behavior and positive habits.

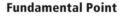

Fundamental Point

It is not the emotion that is judged as good or bad but the behavior that follows the emotion.

- **Delay responding** and above all avoid doing something immediately without thought. These impulsive or reactive behaviors can often be destructive. One way of avoiding acting too quickly is to put on the *brakes* such as putting in a pause, take a breath before responding, walk away, say something like "just a second" and disengage. The intent is to delay responding.

- **Moderate emotions** by following the golden rule—*Don't take things personally.* Recovering alcoholics, especially early in sobriety, have a difficult time in seeing things objectively. It is very easy for them to interpret what is said or done as a personal attack or as "there they go again." For example, Michelle, a recovering alcoholic, is checking some grocery items in the store and someone runs into her with a grocery cart. Michelle could take the incident personally and shout, "Hey. Why don't you watch where you are going? Can't you see I am here?" Or, she could pause and make a nonaggressive or noninflammatory comment such as "Excuse me." If the person apologized, then Michelle would accept the apology. If the person did not apologize, Michelle would let it go, realizing that the person is just not aware. While it is easier said than done, recovering alcoholics must strive over time to view things objectively and not take them personally.

- **Build constructive behavior** by using the practice of *being assertive and not aggressive.* In some instances, an individual is on the receiving end of something said or done which may be quite inappropriate and feedback should be given. The difference in these cases between assertion and aggression is that assertion is a *controlled* or *measured* response, whereas aggression is *reactive* and *confrontational.* For example, someone jumps in front of an individual in line at the post office. The aggressive response might be to get eye-to-eye with the person and shout, "Hey. I was here before you. Who do you think you are? Get down to the end of the line like everyone else," waving a finger in the person's face. An assertive person would approach the person and say calmly and firmly, "Excuse me. We were here before you. There is a line and please go to the end of the line like everyone else." While there are no guarantees what might happen, there is more likelihood that the assertive response would get a better result than the aggressive one. Remember the recommended practice to "Fake it till you make it" while these skills are being established.

- **Build positive habits.** Just as the person who perseverates on negative thoughts and actions will become locked into a negative pattern, the person who dwells on positive thoughts and engages in productive, healthy, and constructive actions will respond that way most of the time. Recovering alcoholics must do all they can to develop good habits, connect with positive people, take care of business at home and at work, and try to lead a quality life. In this way they increase the chances of being able to respond to difficult or challenging situations in appropriate ways regardless of what emotions may arise. They become more and more in control of their own behavior, manage situations with dignity and respect, irrespective of their emotional reactions to circumstances that may come their way.

It is most important for recovering alcoholics to recognize success in managing their behavior following negative emotions. Progress in managing emotions is measured by *what they do* following the experience of emotions rather than what feelings may have emerged.

> **Example A:** The person who becomes angry often becomes aggressive and insults the offender. Good progress is shown when that same person who, on becoming angry, walks away and avoids escalating the situation.

> **Example B:** The person who gets a setback becomes anxious and withdraws to her apartment for two days. The same person, instead of withdrawing, calls a friend, talks about the setback, and comes up with some ideas on how to proceed.

> **Example C:** A recovering alcoholic said someone rammed him with a grocery cart at the store the previous week and he felt a surge of anger and said, "I wanted to shove the guy against the wall and

knock him on his ..." But he didn't. He just continued with his shopping. He then said that he just does not get it that he has been sober for 12 years and he still gets angry. This man should be celebrating instead of feeling down on himself. He was provoked and showed wonderful control by not responding to his anger, letting it go, and continuing with his shopping.

In general, recovering alcoholics must focus on the behaviors they exhibit following the experience of emotions. The goal is to avoid, at all costs, behaviors that are destructive and to exhibit constructive and acceptable behaviors. Finally, it is most important for recovering alcoholics to understand that the full array of emotions may emerge at any time and they must never judge themselves on what emotions occur. Rather, they judge themselves on what they did following the experience of the emotions.

Checklist and Action Plan for Developing Emotional Growth

Form 11.3: Checklist and Action Plan for Developing Emotional Growth, is the fourth checklist and action plan in the series of strategies for assisting recovering alcoholics to obtain growth toward achieving ongoing healthy sobriety. (It follows the checklists and action plans for developing autonomous, cognitive, and social growth, Chapters 8, 9, and 10.)

The instrument, Form 11.3 (Apendix P), begins with listing the prioritized emotions results from Form 11.1 (the positive emotions that need to be developed and the negative ones need to be reduced or controlled). In addition, the operating triggers results from Form 11.2 are listed. The next step is to carefully examine the list of familiar practices for establishing skills to manage emotions productively and to determine which strategies may be workable or not workable for them by selecting *Yes* or *No* in the *Yes/No* column. Since there are several strategies listed for each overall approach, the third column provides space for *Specifics*. In this column the particular aspect of a strategy selected is identified and described as necessary. In the action plan section, the individuals write down the details of how they propose to implement the strategies such as what time of day, location, and with whom they may be engaging in the activity. This checklist and action plan is included in Appendix P: Form 11.3, Checklist and Action Plan for Developing Emotional Growth, and an example is presented in Illustration 11.3.

Background: Continuing with Micheil from Illustrations 11.1 and 11.2

ILLUSTRATION 11.3: Checklist and Action Plan for Developing Emotional Growth

Prioritized Emotions from Form 11.1		Operating Triggers from Form 11.2
1. *Peaceful* 2. *Grateful*	3. *Depressed* 4. *Anxious*	1. *Thoughts* 2. *Communication* 3. *Unresolved conflicts*

Strategies	Selection (Underline) Yes or No	Specifics
1. Maintain initial strategies for obtaining sobriety	<u>Yes</u> No	*I need to refresh my action plans.*
2. Utilize strategies for developing autonomous growth	Yes <u>No</u>	*Okay here.*
3. Utilize strategies for developing cognitive growth	Yes <u>No</u>	*Okay here.*
4. Utilize strategies for developing social growth	<u>Yes</u> No	*This area is huge for me and I will resume my original action plans.*
5. Engage in service activities	Yes <u>No</u>	*I do a lot of service already with AA and will continue.*
6. Manage the triggers for negative emotions	<u>Yes</u> No	*Must address negative thoughts.*
7. Manage the triggers for positive emotions	<u>Yes</u> No	*Must cultivate, these especially gratitude.*
8. Use coping skills for triggers	<u>Yes</u> No	*Must speak my mind early.*
9. Enhance positive emotions	<u>Yes</u> No	*Keep building joy and address gratitude especially to family.*
10. Reduce destructive negative thoughts	<u>Yes</u> No	*Especially related to depression.*
11. Increase constructive positive thoughts	<u>Yes</u> No	*I need to work on this especially looking at the good things in my family.*
12. Adopt meditation practice	<u>Yes</u> No	*This would be new for me but worth a try perhaps.*
13. Establish replacement behaviors	<u>Yes</u> No	*I need to work on this especially in doing more fun things with my family.*
14. Other	Yes <u>No</u>	

ILLUSTRATION 11.3 *Continued*

ACTION PLAN

There is so much to do that I could easily get overwhelmed. My sponsor and I decided I will work on the following:

1. *Meet with sponsor weekly and call daily for a while.*

2. *Develop specific problem solving-plans especially around failure to communicate. I will write things down more.*

3. *Get back to my "to-do" list as it worked for me with initial sobriety. Now I will expand it.*

4. *Find an AA group that focuses on the 11th step and engages in meditation.*

5. *Schedule weekend activities with entire family.*

6. *Spend time after dinner with family.*

7. *Make a concerted effort to switch to positive thoughts when I am dwelling on negative thoughts.*

Chapter Summary

While recovering alcoholics have made commendable gains in becoming sober, they still have much to accomplish toward achieving healthy sobriety. Dealing with and managing emotions is a huge challenge. During the period of alcoholism, individuals used alcohol to avoid meeting their emotional needs. These needs were suppressed. Now that the individuals have accomplished sobriety, these same emotional needs resurface along with the side effects from sustained repression of emotions. It is little wonder that Bill W. in the twilight of his career made this telling comment:

> I think many oldsters who have put AA "booze cure" to severe but successful tests still find that they lack emotional sobriety. Perhaps they will be the spearhead of the next major development in AA. (*The Language of the Heart*, p. 236)

Addressing "emotional sobriety" has been the focus of this chapter. Emotions are easy to notice but hard to define or manage. Emotions themselves fall into a vast array of examples and nuances. To limit this scope and to provide a focus for recovering alcoholics, the well-known text Alcoholics Anonymous was used to identify emotions commonly spoken of regarding alcoholics and recovering alcoholics. Counts were made for the most frequently cited emotions in the text and a list developed reflecting the most common citings. A list was developed to assist recovering alcoholics identify the most prevalent emotions, both positive and negative, operating currently in their lives. This assessment provides the target emotions for strategies designed to promote emotional growth.

One reason that emotions are difficult to manage is that they belong to an interplay of several variables which were described in terms of a cycle of emotions involving six interconnected factors: *triggers, emotions, physiology, thinking, behaviors,* and *impact.* In order to manage emotions, it is argued that three of these factors can be directly manipulated as an intervention—triggers, thinking, and behavior. Strategies are described as to how these factors can be manipulated to control the impact of emotions.

These measures taken to develop emotional growth, along with steps taken to assure autonomous, cognitive, and social growth, set the stage for recovering alcoholics to make solid gains toward healthy and productive sobriety in their lives.

SECTION FOUR

Additional Considerations

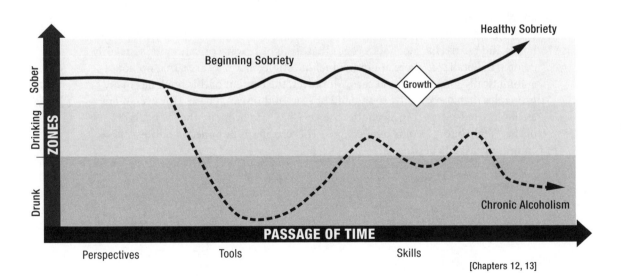

The first three sections of this book (Section One: Critical Perspectives; Section Two: Tools for Beginning Sobriety; Section Three: Skills for Healthy Sobriety) are written as a progression from understanding alcoholism and committing to becoming sober, to maintaining sobriety, and to achieving a better and healthier lifestyle. Each section, to this point, leads to the next section and each chapter sets the stage for subsequent chapters. However, this last section, Section Four: Additional Considerations, is different because the content lies *outside* of this progression.

Chapter 12, Addressing Relapses *as Needed*, addresses issues related to *relapse*, that is, the recovering alcoholic begins to drink again. Ideally this situation should not arise as the first eleven chapters are designed to help alcoholics and their service providers understand the nature of alcoholism and take steps to achieve and maintain sobriety. However, reality tells us that many recovering alcoholics begin to drink again and develop a revolving lifestyle of sobriety and relapse. Details are presented in this chapter to help recovering alcoholics prevent relapse and to recover should relapse occur.

Chapter 13, Frequently Asked Questions, is the other chapter that falls outside of the progression from alcoholism to healthy sobriety. Chapters 1–11 are designed in a logical order with clear-cut and independent chapters. These earlier chapters address alcoholics and recovering alcoholics in general with a reasonable attempt to cover the range of application. However, it is understood that life for many alcoholics and recovering alcoholics is not that straightforward or cannot be so readily compartmentalized. There are individual questions that may arise that do not fit automatically into the general case. Moreover, the content of this book has many principles that are basically sound and have a solid research base. However, many alcoholics and recovering alcoholics are very likely to bring up the "What if ..." or the "Yeah, but ..." kinds of questions. This chapter is designed to address these commonly asked questions.

Addressing Relapses as Needed

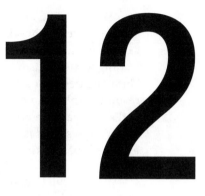

*One must exercise proper deliberation, plan carefully before making a move,
and be alert in guarding against relapse following a renaissance.*

– Horace

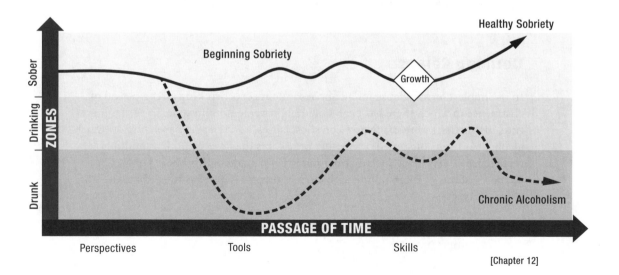

I n Sections Two and Three, detailed information has been presented on procedures for breaking the cycle of alcoholism and developing skills for lifelong, healthy sobriety. Essentially, two paths have been described, one leading to alcoholism and the other, the ideal path, leading to healthy sobriety. Unfortunately, not all alcoholics follow these paths so cleanly. Many alcoholics resume drinking and disrupt their path to sobriety. Then they become sober and start again. In effect, these alcoholics, in their quest for sobriety, experience relapses, that is, periods of drinking and starting over before they finally become sober. In these cases, relapses become part of their pathway to sobriety.

It is very difficult to understand how an individual can endure the personal turmoil associated with the process of detoxification and make the demanding initial steps to become sober only to start drinking again. This phenomenon, known as relapse, would be easier to accommodate if it were an irregular event or the exception. It is not. It has been widely reported that up to *90 percent* of alcoholics experience at least one relapse following treatment (Witkiewitz & Marlatt, 2009; Polivy & Herman, 2002). This number is staggering. How can so many alcoholics return to something so self-destructive after they experience some level of success with recovery?

The purpose of this chapter is to examine the issues related to this confounding question and to carefully consider what can be done programmatically, both short term and long term, to significantly reverse this trend. The topics addressed are: 1. Defining relapse, 2. Identifying contributing factors, 3. Preventing relapses, 4. Strategies for recovering from a relapse, and 5. Checklist and action plan.

Defining Relapse

In its simplest form, relapse for alcoholics is defined as drinking after a period of abstinence in which there has been noted improvement in lifestyle. In earlier literature, distinctions were made between slips, lapses, and relapses based on how much alcohol has been consumed or whether or not it is the first, second, or multiple recurrence of drinking. Such distinctions are not made in this book. For the purposes of this chapter, in line with current usage, relapse has these three defining characteristics:

- Any recurrence of drinking (whether it be the first time, second time, or multiple times)

- Any level of consumption of alcohol (whether it be one or two glasses or an all-night binge)

- The return to drinking follows a period of abstinence and improvement in lifestyle. This factor excludes those who have an ongoing cycle of drinking and quitting for short periods of time (this pattern is better described as a form of alcoholism rather than relapse).

In Figure 12.1, Relapse, two pathways are depicted. The solid line shows the pathway dipping into the *Drinking* and *Drunk* zones following a period of sobriety. This pathway indicates that the individual has started to drink again (pathway to alcoholism). The broken lines show that the pathway leading to healthy sobriety has been disrupted. The box labeled "Relapse" is at the junction between the two pathways located in the *Sober* zone following *Beginning Sobriety* period. This indicates that the relapse process starts while the individual is in a state of sobriety but not healthy sobriety (and as we shall see later in this chapter, that the process of relapse starts well before the first drink is taken).

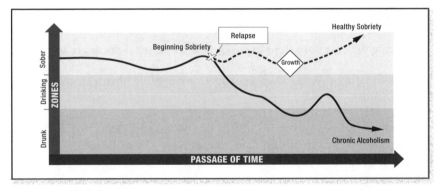

FIGURE 12.1: Relapse

Identifying Contributing Factors

Relapse is a complex issue with several contributing and interacting causes. The major contributing factors consist of: a. Treating relapse as part of recovery, b. The nature of addiction and disease, c. Interacting effects of alcoholism, d. Inadequate planning in the first place, e. Abandonment of effective practices, f. Need to test the waters, g. Reinforcement–extinction cycle, h. Managing surprises and extenuating circumstances, i. Edging closer to former haunts and routines, and j. Seeking just cause.

Treating Relapse as Part of Recovery

It may be that some practitioners and recovering alcoholics view relapse as an inevitable part of the recovery process. In other words, individuals must go through the cycle of abstinence from alcohol then relapse before sobriety can really be attained. In effect, relapse is viewed as an integral part of the recovery process. This recovery model is akin to a *two-steps-forward-and-one step-back process* approach.

The approach taken in this book is that if relapse is expected, then there is the danger of setting up a *self-fulfilling prophecy*. While statistics indicate that relapse is very common, steps can be taken to reduce the incidence of relapse such as:

- ensuring an ongoing firm commitment to recover

- taking necessary precautions to abstain from alcohol

- taking the necessary steps to ensure unmet personal needs are addressed

- ensuring appropriate levels of support are in place (themes throughout this book)

The situation is analogous to car accidents. Just because accidents frequently occur, it does not mean we have to accept them as inevitable. We still must do what we can to reduce the incidence of car accidents.

Finally, when relapse is viewed as part of recovery, many alcoholics may recover while some may not. The sad reality is that some of these individuals may not have been lost to alcoholism if recovery was presented to them in a way that prevented relapse rather than accommodated it. Gjesvold (2011) reported a significant finding related to services offered by Serenity Lane (a residential program for alcoholics in Oregon). Specifically, that persons who had undergone treatment at the program could receive accommodation and treatment free of charge, Friday through Sunday, if they relapsed. The finding was that the incidence of relapses *soared*.

The Nature of Addiction and Disease

While there is some dispute in the field as to whether alcoholism is a disease or not, one position is clear—alcoholism is one powerful addiction. Perhaps Gorski and Miller (1986) described the problem best by adopting the term "addiction-disease." Regardless of the nomenclature, the potential for relapse among recovering alcoholics in practice is no different than for those with chronic diseases such as diabetes, asthma, and hypertension. Relapse can occur at any time irrespective of the number of years of sobriety. Similarly, just as individuals who suffer from chronic diseases must adjust their lifestyles and constantly take charge of their own care, so do recovering alcoholics, otherwise relapse will most likely occur.

Interacting Effects of Alcoholism

The far-reaching systemic effects of alcoholism were addressed in Chapters 1, 2, 6, and all of Section Three. It is difficult to isolate the effects of alcoholism not only because of the long-term effects, but these effects interact with each other.

Gorski and Miller (1986) in their landmark book on relapse, *Staying Sober,* coined the phrase *bio-psycho-social damage* to capture the interacting issues recovering alcoholics experience from alcoholism with respect to physical health (bio-), mental health (psycho-) and relationships with others (social-). These authors noted that comprehensive interventions need to be developed to address this three-fold interaction. Unless such all-inclusive detail is systematically addressed, the recovering alcoholic will be vulnerable to relapse.

Inadequate Planning in the First Place

Probably, the most across-the-board reason for recovering alcoholics to return to drinking is the failure to understand that there is more to becoming sober than just *abstinence from alcohol.* A recovering alcoholic has many personal needs that must be planned for in the areas of *autonomous, cognitive, social,* and *emotional* growth (see Section Three, Chapters 8, 9, 10, and 11). If these personal needs are not effectively addressed, the recovering alcoholic will most likely function as the classic *dry drunk* who is sober but displays all of the maladjusted behaviors exhibited when drinking. It is totally naïve to think that all alcoholics have to do is quit drinking and put all of their efforts into avoiding drinking, in order to remain sober. Wrong!

A comprehensive intervention plan must begin in the commitment period prior to becoming sober and systematically adjusted throughout the individual's life. The plan has two focuses: first, to *sustain abstinence* from drinking alcohol, and second to develop, implement, and *maintain ongoing personal growth*. Failure to accommodate both of these components will most surely result in relapse.

Abandonment of Effective Practices

When recovering alcoholics quit drinking they experience many benefits through becoming sober, such as feeling better in the morning, looking better, eating better, being able to do other things that are enjoyable instead of drinking, and being more productive at work. Unfortunately, these success experiences give some individuals a false sense of security. They begin to feel somewhat triumphant because they have struggled with alcoholism and begin to slowly drop the very practices that enabled them to become sober and remain sober. For example, they stop seeing their support person or sponsor and may stop going to meetings. They begin to take risks and nudge closer to the old routines they had when they were drinking. In a sense they feel they have been cured. They think that alcoholism is a disease and that they have been cured. Clearly, with this attitude or belief system, it will not be long before they begin drinking and suffer a relapse. While individuals may eventually wean themselves of the supports used in beginning sobriety, it is critical that this process does not occur too early or too abruptly.

Need to Test the Waters of Drinking in Moderation

Recovering alcoholics are keenly aware of the many sacrifices they have to make in order to become and remain sober. For example, they stay away from old haunts and friends, feel different at parties and gatherings because others are drinking and they are not, and have to establish many competing routines such as going for walks instead of going to a happy hour event. The question often arises for a recovering alcoholic: "Is there a chance now since I have broken the habit of drinking that I may be able to drink in moderation?" or "I don't want to get drunk, but it sure would be nice if I could just have a couple. I wonder if I could do that." Some individuals would firmly say, along with their support person or sponsor, that there is no way of being moderate. There is no middle ground when it comes to addictions or the disease of alcoholism. If you start up then you will become an alcoholic again. Or, they are told that it is far easier to abstain from alcohol rather than drink in moderation. However, some recovering alcoholics may not be satisfied with these warnings. They want to know firsthand. They may even know someone who quit drinking and is now able to drink in moderation.

If individuals proceed with *testing the waters*, some criteria need to be firmly set in place and understood *before* they start drinking. Critical criteria include questions like, "Can you predetermine how many drinks you will have and stick to it?" Also, they need to monitor how often they drink. They may start out drinking once a week on Fridays, for example. However, it is not long before they are finding reasons to drink every other day and so on.

Alcoholics need to understand that alcoholism is an addiction or, if you like, an addiction-disease. For the vast majority of recovering alcoholics, drinking in moderation is not an option and that a return to drinking is a return to alcoholism with all its very serious harmful outcomes.

Reinforcement–Extinction Cycle

This behavioral paradigm of the reinforcement–extinction cycle can come into play regarding the relationship between alcoholism, recovery, and relapse. Typically when individuals begin to break a habit, especially a self-destructive one such as weight control, smoking, and alcoholism, relatives and friends are highly likely to make many positive comments and provide encouragement and attention in the early stages on how good the person looks and so on. This high level of attention is usually very *reinforcing* to the individual making the effort to bring about important changes in their lives in becoming sober. However, after some time, the attention, encouragement, and positive comments from others begin to fade as they get used to seeing the individual in this condition of sobriety. The recovery no longer attains comment, which puts the individual on *extinction* (the reinforcement has been withdrawn). Some individuals may then return to their former self-destructive habits, begin drinking again—relapse, which is noticed by friends and families causing them renewed concern. Now if the individual quits drinking again and becomes sober, the attention is renewed by friends and family, perhaps at a higher level than before because they do not want the individual to return to the self-destructive habit of alcoholism. Now, the recovering alcoholics have learned that through relapse they can restore even higher levels of attention, encouragement, and positive comments upon renewed abstinence. A reinforcement–extinction cycle has been established. Naturally, there would be a limit before friends and family give up, but meanwhile the recovering alcoholic has found an effective way to control and maintain attention from friends and family (at least for some time). Clearly, the recovering alcoholic needs to establish intrinsic reinforcement, importance of what sobriety means to the recovering alcoholic rather than rely of extrinsic reinforcement gained from responses by others.

Managing Surprises and Extenuating Circumstances

In some cases recovering alcoholics become quite firm with their ability to maintain sobriety in their regular daily routines. However, on some occasions something out of the ordinary arises which has not occurred during the individual's sobriety to this point, such as a visit from a longtime friend from overseas; a promotion and solid raise in employment; or birth of a first child. Similarly, sudden circumstances could be downers, such as loss of a job, death in the family, or serious injury. The recovering alcoholic has not practiced sobriety under these conditions and quickly associates drinking with these occasions and how much the drink would enhance the situation. The recovering alcoholic may also argue that a drink under these conditions should not be a problem because these situations occur only rarely. However, once individuals start drinking, for whatever the reason, they are likely to continue because of the nature of their addiction to alcohol.

Fundamental Rule

Under no circumstances should a recovering alcoholic return to drinking.

Edging Closer to Former Haunts and Routines

Once recovering alcoholics become sober and are able to maintain sobriety for some time, they may drop their guard in avoiding the places and occasions where they used to drink. They may assume that they have their drinking under control and it will not matter if they visit their old haunts and make contact with their former drinking buddies. For many recovering alcoholics this would be a trap and set the stage for a relapse. Recovering alcoholics have to make the firm resolve that this is not for them and that they need to establish new routines and new friends or meet their old friends under different circumstance such as having breakfast or a midmorning coffee. They do not have to meet at a bar. It is also important to accept the reality that drinking buddies of recovering alcoholics will continue to meet in their bars or watering holes with or without them.

Seeking Just Cause

It is not unusual for recovering alcoholics to really have their hearts set on drinking again but they do not want to appear as though that is their plan. They are looking for an excuse. They are looking for something else to arise so they can justify their drinking with thoughts such as "How could I refuse a drink under these circumstances" or "Anyone is entitled to a drink under these conditions." The reality is that these individuals have already made up their minds to drink again and are looking for a justifiable reason to drink.

Preventing Relapses

Preventing relapses is an integral part of the process for becoming sober. Recovering alcoholics must understand that alcoholism is a powerful addiction, or addiction-disease, and simply abstaining from alcohol is not sufficient to curb the cravings for alcohol and manage the many harmful effects that arise from alcoholism (such as autonomous, cognitive, social, and emotional impairments). In many respects the recovering alcoholic is a *damaged* person so that many ongoing steps are needed during recovery to address this personal damage.

In effect, the key to preventing relapse is for the recovering alcoholic to make a firm commitment to *doing whatever it takes* to not only remain sober (Chapter 3), but to making a life commitment to doing what it takes to meet the personal needs of the individual described in Chapters 7, 8, 9, 10, and 11. Individuals need to be reminded of the necessity for this commitment as early as the detoxification step (Chapter 4) and frequently during subsequent stages of recovery (Chapters 5–11). It cannot be overemphasized that recovery is a long process requiring ongoing effort and commitment to abstain from alcohol and to address personal needs, otherwise relapse is inevitable.

Strategies for Recovering from a Relapse

Unfortunately a relapse will occur for some individuals even given every effort has been made to prevent relapse (the focus of the majority of the content in this book). It seems *two steps forward and one step back* is to be their process for recovery. It is most important for recovering alcoholics to understand that relapse is not the end of the world and that they should not give up on themselves. When a relapse occurs, there are usually four steps required for the recovery process to be resumed: a. Pinpointing the contributing factor(s), b. Implementing strategies to address contributing factors, c. Starting over, and d. Resuming an ongoing life plan for abstinence and personal growth.

Pinpointing the Contributing Factor(s)

Before individuals attempt to resume recovery from a relapse, it is very important to determine the reasons why the relapse occurred. If these pinpoints are not made, there is a high likelihood that another relapse will occur because these reasons were not specifically addressed. Several factors were identified in a previous section of this chapter which will serve as a checklist for determining the operative factors for the individual's relapse. The factors are listed in Box 12.1: Factors Contributing to Relapse. The idea is for recovering alcoholics to examine each factor in the list and assess whether or not the factor played a role in leading to the relapse. It is strongly recommended that this assessment is conducted by the recovering alcoholic in conjunction with a support person or sponsor. The reason is that the information reported by the recovering alcoholic may not be reliable. Alcoholics are often in denial regarding information related to their drinking patterns. Consequently, when they begin the recovery process from relapse they may resort to denial practices. A second opinion, or reliability check, is essential to obtaining accurate pinpoints on factors contributing to the individual's relapse.

Once the pinpoints have been made, recovering alcoholics are then encouraged, with their support person or sponsor, to select specific strategies for managing these identified factors.

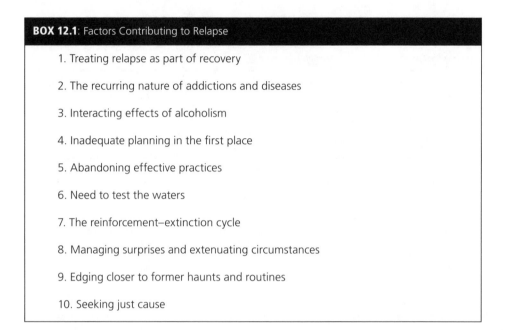

BOX 12.1: Factors Contributing to Relapse

1. Treating relapse as part of recovery

2. The recurring nature of addictions and diseases

3. Interacting effects of alcoholism

4. Inadequate planning in the first place

5. Abandoning effective practices

6. Need to test the waters

7. The reinforcement–extinction cycle

8. Managing surprises and extenuating circumstances

9. Edging closer to former haunts and routines

10. Seeking just cause

Implementing Strategies to Address Contributing Factors

Once the individuals have pinpointed the factors contributing to their relapse, the next step is to design strategies that specifically target these factors. This book is replete with strategies for addressing the major aspects of recovery from alcoholism. Individuals are strongly encouraged to select strategies that were helpful to them in the beginning phases of their sobriety (especially working with a support person and attending meetings). These strategies coupled with more precise strategies for addressing the factors leading to the relapse should help individuals resume their efforts toward more permanent states of sobriety.

In Box 12.2, Contributing Factors and Strategies for Addressing Relapse, the ten factors leading to relapse are listed along with some corresponding general approaches for addressing these factors. Recovering alcoholics, and their support persons, are encouraged to examine these strategies and develop specific variations for adoption in the Checklist and Action Plan for Preventing Relapse (Form 12.1, Appendix Q) addressed later in this chapter.

BOX 12.2: Contributing Factors and Strategies for Addressing Relapse	
Contributing Factors	**Strategies**
1. Treating relapse as part of recovery	This is a mistake. The goal is sustained sobriety and excludes any thought or occurrence of relapse. If relapse happens then is must be dealt with but certainly not planned for.
2. The recurring nature of addictions and diseases	Fully understand that alcoholism, as with other addictions and diseases always has the potential to recur.
3. Interacting effects of alcoholism	Fully understand that there are several very serious effects of alcoholism that impact severely on the body, the brain, the mind, and social and emotional areas. These effects are linked and intervention must target all areas.
4. Inadequate planning in the first place	Planning has to begin with becoming free from alcohol right through to a sober lifestyle. Complete planning for all stages is necessary.
5. Abandoning effective practices	Recovering alcoholics must commit to maintaining the critical practices throughout initial sobriety (such as working with a sponsor and attending meetings).
6. Need to test the waters	Realize that the chances of becoming a moderate drinker are very slim. Put in safeguards to return immediately to beginning sobriety steps if this direction is pursued.
7. Reinforcement–extinction cycle	Here the individual's motivation becomes dependent on external reinforcement (praise and attention from others). Steps must be taken to develop intrinsic or personal motivation.
8. Managing surprises and extenuating circumstances	Seriously. Drinking under any circumstances is not an option.
9. Edging closer to former haunts and routines	This is a commitment issue. The individual must commit to doing what it takes to remain sober and studiously avoid whatever threatens sobriety.
10. Seeking just cause	Again this is a commitment issue. Individuals must commit for lifetime healthy sobriety. Any leaning toward drinking or seeking reasons to drink is an aberration from this commitment.

Starting Over

In conjunction with addressing the factors that may have led to the relapse, individuals now face the task of having to become sober again. Essentially it is starting over except this time around the individuals will need to have firmer resolve and be more vigilant in following the procedures to become sober and remain sober. The extent of the treatment to regain sobriety depends on the length of time the individual has been in the relapse phase, the level of drinking during relapse, and the individual's alcoholic history. Typically, the treatment begins with detoxification (Chapter 4), followed by, or in conjunction with, management of cravings (Chapter 5), and then the steps for managing the initial needs of beginning sobriety (Chapter 6). The recovering alcoholic in relapse is encouraged, with assistance from a support person, to re-examine earlier action plans for each of these stages and to add or modify strategies in the action plan to recover from the relapse. The general references to this text for establishing initial sobriety are presented in Box 12.3: References to Achieving Initial Sobriety.

BOX 12.3: References to Achieving Initial Sobriety

Step	Chapter Reference	Form Reference
Step 1: Renew Commitment	Chapter 3: Making a Commitment	Form 3.2: Checklist and Action Plan for Making a Commitment to Quit Alcohol
Step 2: Detoxification	Chapter 4: Detoxification	Selection of specific detoxification plan. Development of short term exit plan.
Step 3: Manage Cravings	Chapter 5: Defusing Cravings	Form 5.1: Checklist and Action Plan for Cravings
Step 4: Manage beginning sobriety	Chapter 6: Meeting Initial Needs	Form 6.1: Checklist and Action Plan for Initial Needs

Resuming an Ongoing Lifeplan for Abstinence and Personal Growth

At this juncture the recovering alcoholic has pinpointed what factors have contributed to his or her relapse, developed and implemented strategies for addressing these factors, and resumed practicing successful strategies for beginning sobriety. It is especially important for the recovering alcoholic to take every precaution to ensure that relapse does not recur. A cycle of sobriety-relapse is a common form of alcoholism and must be avoided. The recovering alcoholic has already demonstrated that he or she can do what it takes to attain beginning sobriety. Once individuals

have attained a solid base of sobriety this next time around and have reliably implemented strategies to effectively address their needs at this beginning sobriety level,
the next step is to target long-term healthy sobriety. The step involves targeting
the personal growth areas (autonomous, cognitive, social, and emotional) the
subject area of Section Three (Chapters 7–11). The general references to this text for
addressing long-term personal growth areas are presented in Box 12.4: References to
Achieving Lifelong Healthy Sobriety.

BOX 12.4: References to Achieving Lifelong Healthy Sobriety		
Personal Growth Area	**Chapter Reference**	**Form Reference**
Autonomous Growth	Chapter 7: Key considerations for personal growth Chapter 8 Skills for *Autonomous Growth*	Forms 8.1, 8.2, 8.3, and 8.4 (Appendices E, F, G, and H)
Cognitive Growth	Chapter 9 Skills for *Cognitive Growth*	Forms 9.1and 9.2 (Appendices I and J)
Social Growth	Chapter 10: Skills for *Social Growth*	Forms 10.1, 10.2, and 10.3 (Appendices K, L, and M)
Emotional Growth	Chapter 11: Skills for *Emotional Growth*	Form 11.1 (Appendix N)

Checklist and Action Plan for Preventing Future Relapse

The checklist and action plan for the recovering alcoholic in relapse in many ways is not that much different from the plan for the alcoholic who is about to quit drinking for the first time. The obvious difference is that the individual in relapse has already quit at least once. The planning differences are that the recovering alcoholics, now in relapse, must pinpoint the factors that contributed to their resumption of drinking and use strategies to prevent further recurrences of drinking. The additional layers now are measures to be taken to address the relapse otherwise the recovery plan is the same as for addressing alcoholism (detoxification, managing cravings, using strategies for beginning sobriety and long-term healthy sobriety).

In Form 12.1, Checklist and Action Plan for Preventing Future Relapse, individuals who have experienced a relapse rate each of ten factors that may have contributed to the relapse. Each factor is judged *Yes* (applicable) or *No* (not applicable). It is recommended that these judgments are made by the alcoholic in relapse in conjunction with a support person or sponsor so as to obtain more reliable measures. The ratings are then summarized according the scores of *Yes* or *No*. An action plan is then developed in which interventions are selected targeting the factors scored *Yes*. Once this action plan is completed, recovering alcoholics will need to progress through each of the stages for recovery once again—detoxification (Chapter 4), managing cravings (Chapter 5), managing initial needs of beginning sobriety (Chapter 6), and planning for long-term healthy sobriety (Chapters 7–11). In revisiting these steps recovering alcoholics in relapse are encouraged, with assistance from a support person, to re-examine earlier action plans for each of these stages and to add or modify strategies in the action plan to recover from the relapse. A blank form is presented in Appendix Q: Form 12.1, Checklist and Action Plan for Preventing Future Relapses, and an example appears as Illustration 12.1. Recovering alcoholics are then directed to the chapters on tools (Chapters 4–6) and the chapters on skills (Chapters 7–11) to start the process over for regaining and maintaining sobriety and for developing lifelong healthy sobriety.

Background: Elaine, a 45-year-old married woman with 26 months of sobriety, was laid off the previous year and has been concerned with finding another position. She devoted most of the last 6 months to job searching as an office manager and has been unsuccessful. She is adamant that she will not accept just any job. She wants something somewhat close to her qualifications and experience. She has noticed that she has had numerous arguments with her spouse, children, members of her church, and members of the Recovery Fellowship to which she belongs. Her sponsor, who has worked with Elaine from the beginning of her sobriety, confronted her and said that she was on a "dry drunk" roll and that she was headed for a relapse. Elaine denied this, got angry and left the meeting abruptly. After several months had passed Elaine called her sponsor and said that she had just gotten out of detox following a series of passing out incidents from drinking. She wanted to try again.

ILLUSTRATION 12.1: Checklist and Action Plan for Preventing Future Relapse

Contributing Factors to Relapse	Applicability Rating (Underline) Yes: Applicable No: Not applicable	General Strategies (from Box 12.2)
1. Treating relapse as part of recovery	Yes <u>No</u>	Avoid relapse at all costs with a comprehensive recovery plan.
2. The nature of addictions and disease	Yes <u>No</u>	Re-examine alcoholism as an addiction-disease.
3. Interacting effects of alcoholism	Yes <u>No</u>	Re-examine the damaging effects of alcoholism.
4. Inadequate planning in the first place	Yes <u>No</u>	Develop a comprehensive plan from quitting to healthy sobriety.
5. Abandonment of effective practices	<u>Yes</u> No	Pick up previously used effective practices following detoxification.
6. Need to test the waters	Yes <u>No</u>	Avoid this at all costs. But if insistent ensure full return to recovery plan if problems arise.
7. Reinforcement–extinction cycle	Yes <u>No</u>	Recognize the role of support from others but fully invest in your own efforts.
8. Managing surprises or extenuating circumstances	<u>Yes</u> No	There are no exceptions. Never take a drink.
9. Edging closer to former haunts and routines	Yes <u>No</u>	Make a firm resolve to avoid situations where drinking is likely.
10. Seeking just cause	<u>Yes</u> No	Recognize this is denial. Make the firm resolve to quit and stay sober.

ILLUSTRATION 12.1 *Continued*

SUMMARY

Factors scored Yes:
Underline and total: <u>1</u> 2 3 4 <u>5</u> 6 7 <u>8</u> 9 <u>10</u>   Total Yes: <u> 4 </u>

Factors scored No: Total No: <u> 6 </u>

ACTION PLAN (Select strategies to match the contributing factors scored Yes).

Factor 1: Treating relapse as part of recovery

a. *Find new sponsor who is very aggressive in planning so relapse will not occur.*

b. *In initial meeting develop new plan.*

Factor 5: Abandonment of effective practices

a. *New plan developed with sponsor stipulates weekly meetings and bi-weekly check-ins with sponsor as for beginning sobriety stage.*

b. *Resume weekly AA meetings.*

c. *Resume journal writing and addressing anger management with sponsor.*

Factor 8: Managing surprises or extenuating circumstances

a. *Establish with sponsor the absolute hard rule that under no circumstance will drinking occur.*

b. *Identify times or places when drinking might occur and develop avoidance plan.*

Factor 10: Seeking just cause

In journaling and meeting with sponsor discuss when and where denial occurs and plan alternative responses.

Chapter Summary

One of the most disturbing aspects of treatment and recovery for alcoholics is the very high rate of relapse where individuals return to drinking following a period of sobriety. A number of factors have been reported for contributing to the return to drinking. Foremost is the erroneous and misleading belief that relapse is an *inevitable* part of the recovery process. Once it is accepted that relapse can be prevented with careful planning, two of the most central factors contributing to relapse are: a *lack of firm resolve* to quit drinking and systematic *abandonment of practices* that helped the individual achieve sobriety. The various factors are described in detail and corresponding interventions outlined for preventing further relapses.

Perhaps the most important point for recovering alcoholics in regard to understanding why they are vulnerable to relapse is that maintaining sobriety requires more than just *abstinence* from alcohol use. Long-term sobriety requires a plan involving *both* abstinence from alcohol use and ongoing efforts to ensure that personal growth areas (autonomous, cognitive, social, and emotional) are addressed. Alcoholism has caused substantial brain damage to individuals along with accompanying impairments in physical, mental, social, and psychological health. Abstinence from alcohol will not take care of these needs by itself. What is needed is a comprehensive lifelong plan designed to incorporate both abstinence and personal growth. The earlier chapters in this book describe the details for such plans.

A checklist and action plan is described to assist the recovering alcoholic to pinpoint factors contributing to the relapse and strategies for preventing further occurrences. The recovering alcoholic is then encouraged to revisit earlier checklists and action plans for establishing beginning sobriety and then proceed in developing and sustaining an uninterrupted lifelong healthy sobriety.

Frequently Asked Questions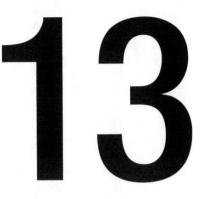

The most erroneous stories are those we think we know best —
and therefore never scrutinize or question.

— Stephen Jay Gould

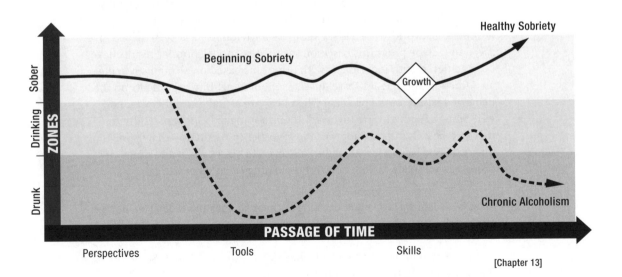

A book such as this is typically designed to take the major building blocks of content and develop the material into discrete chapters. The division and flow of the content is chosen to suit the logic of the approach and the development of the content. Sometimes questions arise that do not fit so simply into these arbitrary chapter divisions or that may overlap with several chapters. In some cases questions arise as individuals think through some content and perceive that the content does not go far enough for them. The purpose of this chapter is to address some of the common questions that arise in dealing with the nature of alcoholism and its ongoing treatment. Where possible responses to these questions will be based directly on the content of this book or derived from the basic principles underlying the book. Each question is simply cited followed by a response.

1. **Is alcoholism a disease or not? I am confused. I hear heated arguments sometimes about this at meetings.**

   Yes the field is divided on the subject of whether alcoholism is a disease or not. The American Medical Association, most insurance companies, and the world-wide treatment program Alcoholics Anonymous (AA) view it as a disease. Other professionals and programs such as Rational Emotive Therapy view it primarily as a self-inflicted addiction.

   The bottom line is that there is presumably total agreement that alcoholism is a staggering health issue causing crises to many individuals and their families on a world-wide basis. Countless individuals have been helped, lives saved in fact, by programs based on the disease model. Similar results have been achieved with individuals with programs based on alcoholism being an addiction and not a disease. It seems moot to get into arguments on the perceived nature of the problem when lives are at stake and the personal well-being of so many are involved. If one approach helps some individuals—so be it. If another approach helps other individuals—that is fine too. The real issue is whether alcoholics receive the kind of help and interventions that are likely to be successful in helping them recover.

2. **What is alcoholism? I can quit drinking at times so does this mean I am not an alcoholic?**

   There are many interpretations of what alcoholism is or is not. Some think it is based on whether or not a person can exercise any control over their drinking. For example, an individual decides to quit drinking two days and is successful. Many individuals put in various controls such as drinking on alternate days, only drinking certain kinds of alcohol, limiting when to start drinking and so on. All of these practices are variations of control. The most widely used definition or indicator of whether a person is an alcoholic or not lies in whether or not the *person can stop drinking after they start*. In other words, can they set a limit on their drinking and stick to that limit? If they can then, they are probably not alcoholic. Typically, the alcoholic cannot stop drinking, once they begin regardless of other controls they may exert such as when they start drinking. Basically, once they start drinking they keep drinking till they pass out, or have to go home, or until they run out of alcohol. If alcohol is available they will keep drinking. The alcohol takes over. This is alcoholism in practice.

3.   **What is the difference between alcohol abuse and alcohol dependence?**

In general terms alcoholic dependence is associated with alcoholism where individuals cannot control their drinking. They are unable to stop drinking after they start. Alcohol abuse, on the other hand, is used to describe individuals who can control their drinking but who decide to drink excessively, to the point of getting drunk, on certain occasions. The difference lies in the word control. Alcohol dependence implies lack of control over drinking while alcohol abuse implies control over drinking. With alcohol dependence it is the alcohol that controls the person's drinking. With alcohol abuse, it is the individual who controls the drinking. It is important to note that alcohol abuse can lead to alcohol dependence as well which means that alcohol itself begins to take over control.

4.   **How do I know that I have made an adequate commitment to abstinence?**

You never drink no matter what or how much you want to! This response may seem somewhat flippant given there is serious intent behind the question. Let's face it. Alcoholics have made a serious commitment to drinking, so much so that there is a good chance it will kill them or at least ruin their lives at many levels. This mind-set of continuing to drink no matter what must be reversed. A major reason individuals who quit drinking and then start up again, relapse, is that their commitment to quit is not strong enough. The recovering alcoholic must say never when it comes to drinking and that means *never* under any circumstances.

5.   **Can a person become too dependent on their recovery group or sponsor?**

This question gets at the nature of addiction or displaced addiction. That is, once a person is addicted to alcohol and quits is likely to become addicted to something else such as a recovery group. There is no question that when an alcoholic quits drinking there will be a strong withdrawal period making the individual particularly vulnerable. At this time strong support is needed. This support can come from other individuals such as sponsors and from the fellowship and encouragement provided by recovery groups. It is natural for the recovering alcoholic to experience a strong level of bonding and attachment with a sponsor and recovery groups. Is this relationship dependence? No, not necessarily. The relationship could become unhealthy and perhaps dependent if that was all there was. However, the recovering alcoholic still needs to address what it takes to attain healthy sobriety with careful attention to strategies designed to address the impairments caused by alcoholism and pursue personal growth. So, the recovering alcoholic can greatly benefit from the support from sponsors and recovery groups, especially early in sobriety. Nevertheless, steps must be taken in addition to this level of support to attain a long-term healthy sobriety. In this way the recovering alcoholic will not become dependent upon support groups.

6.   **I have heard that Alcoholics Anonymous is a cult. Is it?**

No. The defining characteristic of a cult is the control the cult exerts over its members to the extent that the thinking and acting of cult members is uniform and dictated usually by the cult leader. Sure AA certainly has passionate and outspoken members who are convinced that the organization has saved their lives, or at least has been significantly influential in helping its members maintain sobriety. As someone once said "It is hard to be objective about something that has saved your life." Moreover, it is well known that there is tremendous diversity and variability in AA groups. Members are encouraged to shop around to find a group that suits them. This kind of diversity would not be found nor tolerated in cults.

7.   **If an alcoholic won't seek help, what can I do?**

This is a hard question because there is no simple answer. A relative or friend sees someone who is clearly drinking excessively, causing significant harm to self and others, and yet persists with drinking. The problem is compounded when the alcoholic becomes abusive toward those who try to help. It is very disturbing to experience the powerlessness and abuse that comes from trying to help an alcoholic. The best advice seems to be to keep trying, to keep making suggestions and requests to address the problem. Who knows when the alcoholic will begin to face up to the problems? Sometimes they have to hit rock bottom such as getting jailed, lose their job, have their spouse leave them, or become seriously ill. Even then some alcoholics do not begin to address their alcoholism. The outsiders, relatives or friends, must not take the rejection of their efforts as a personal failure. Rather, they need to understand the power of this incredibly harmful addiction and keep doing what they can to steer or set the stage for the alcoholic to begin to address the problems. The key is perseverance even under these difficult conditions. Joining support groups for friends or relatives of alcoholics, such as Al-Anon/Alateen , has been helpful to family members adjusting to their loved one's recovery (www.al-anon.alateen.org).

8. **Are certain groups or cultures more likely to become alcoholic than others?**

Yes, definitely. Demographic research has shown that children of alcoholics are particularly prone to drinking at an early age and becoming alcoholics through their lives. Generational alcoholism is quite common unfortunately. Certain cultures, especially those native cultures where alcohol has been introduced late in their people's development coupled with the sudden displacement of their own culture. This has been the sad case with Native North Americans and Aboriginals in Australia. Members of these displaced cultures have serious problems with alcoholism. Individuals who reach retirement age often have problems with alcohol too and become alcoholics because the structures keeping them focused and engaged are no longer present. They have not learned to replace the void with productive alternatives. As the old saying goes: "At retirement the slippers and the bottle come out."

While certain groups are more at risk than others for alcoholism, it must be noted that there is an incredible range in diversity of those who become alcoholics. No group is really spared. Alcoholics can come from the full range of professions; from people with very high intelligence to those much less gifted; across age groups from the very young to the elderly; with those who seem to have everything to those who have nothing or very little; and across gender and sexual orientation. Basically, individuals from any walk of life can become alcoholics.

9.   Why do people continue to drink in spite of all the bad consequences?

The problem with this kind of question is that it is a logical or rational question being applied to an irrational situation. Once an individual becomes an alcoholic it is the effect of alcohol that becomes the driving force for that individual. Needing the drink, having the drink, and experiencing the effect of the drink are all that matter for the alcoholic. Alcoholics develop all sorts of defense mechanisms when it comes to addressing the negative outcomes from drinking no matter how serious such as avoidance, denial, blaming others, oblivion, and flat out lack of interest in these negative effects. Drinking is their only concern and everything else, no matter how serious, becomes quite secondary, if not irrelevant. In some cases the negative effects become the reason for continuing to drink. They get caught up in a vicious circle of drinking causing problems which leads to more drinking which causes more problems and so on.

10. Is beer or wine safer to drink than alcohol?

Drinks that contain less alcohol are obviously safer for the nonalcoholic when one or two drinks are being consumed. The alcohol content of drinks varies considerably. One glass of light beer can have significantly less alcohol content than the same volume of spirits. However, with alcoholics we are not talking about one glass of alcohol! It is the volume of alcohol consumed that matters. One individual can get drunk faster on spirits than another who is drinking beer. The result is the same however. Both individuals became drunk and not able to control how much they drank. The kind of alcohol an alcoholic drinks is not predicated on which drink contains less alcohol. Rather it is simply a matter of taste or which drink they prefer. Some alcoholics switch their drinks and jump around from beer to wine to spirits and so on. Bartenders report that these changeups are a sign the individual is drunk or becoming drunk. In effect the kind of alcohol an alcoholic drinks is irrelevant.

11.   **Why is it that some alcoholics, after a period of abstinence are able to resume drinking in moderation?**

Some individuals consider themselves as alcoholics because they have been drinking quite heavily or with abandon during a period of their lives. They began to drink because of some critical reason and found that they obtained relief from the alcohol and discovered that they enjoyed drinking and perhaps hung out with others who drank heavily and were perceived as alcoholics. Now, for whatever reason, these individuals decide to quit drink and are able to maintain sobriety for a definite period of time. Then they resume drinking and find that they can drink in moderation, that is they can set a reasonable limit on their drinking and keep to the limit. In this sense they are not alcoholics. The working definition used in this book for alcoholism is that the individual cannot predetermine their drinking levels and quit accordingly. Alcoholics, once they begin to drink cannot stop drinking once they have started. They may be able to quit occasionally, but in general once they start they cannot stop. This means that the individuals who can resume drinking after a period of sobriety were not, by this definition, alcoholics in the first place. Simply put they elected to drink heavily, decided to quit, and were able to resume drinking in moderation because they had control over their drinking. They were not alcoholics to begin with.

12.   **What about the role of medications or pharmaceutical interventions during recovery?**

There is no question that prescribed medication has been used successfully in recovery programs for alcoholics and is a prime area of research. The reason it has been barely mentioned in this book is that these authors believe they are not qualified to speak to this subject. The question is a medical question and these authors do not have expertise in the medical field. The approach taken in this book is one of behavioral and skill-based interventions. There is no sense that medical interventions are questioned. Medical interventions play a very important role in ongoing research and treatment of the problem of alcoholism. However, comments or responses to medical related issues belong to qualified medical practitioners. Consequently, if treatment programs use or recommend pharmaceutical interventions, it is assumed that supportive medical expertise is on board and readily available. The simplest suggestion regarding the use of medications and medical interventions in the treatment of alcoholism is the standard response of "Talk to your doctor."

Closing Remarks

*Our goals can only be reached through a vehicle of a plan, in which
we must fervently believe, and upon which we must vigorously act.*
— Pablo Picasso

Alcoholism is unquestionably one of the most far-reaching and long-standing social problems facing not only America but most countries throughout the world. This problem is nondiscriminatory when it comes to age, race, gender, social economic status, educational level, or career orientation. The extent of the concerns are widely known and extensively experienced in all, or most, cultures throughout the world.

It is not as though efforts have been absent in addressing this problem. Alcoholism, its causes and treatment, have been the subject of extensive research at all levels in society including medical, psychological, psychiatric, social, familial, and educational. Similarly, there has been substantial development in practices and approaches to treat the problem based on research, sound theoretical models, and good practice procedures. Community awareness through health programs, church and agency involvement, educational initiatives in schools, media communication, law enforcement, court proceedings, and liquor control regulations, have become quite transparent and very active in endeavors to curtail the problems. However, despite these concerted efforts, which have been of immeasurable help to many individuals, alcoholism is still a major social problem of tragic proportions. The singular statistic, reported in Chapter 1, that the incidence of alcoholism has basically remained unchanged in America over the past decade bears testimony to the depth of the problem and the elusiveness of solutions.

How then can a book like this expect to make any impact on the profound challenge of alcoholism? Clearly, it would be pretentious and offensive to claim that this book has all the answers—that herein lies the solution to this gargantuan issue. Rather, we believe that the content of this book will help some individuals in their endeavors to achieve lifelong sobriety, assist support personnel in their work with recovering alcoholics, and provide a focus for ongoing research and practice on interventions for alcoholism.

Two Perspectives

There are two defining perspectives in this book. First, there is a *behavioral approach* for the analysis of the problem and the design of interventions (tools and skills). This approach has been widely used and documented in effectively addressing serious problem behavior in schools, mental health institutions, and prisons. The behavioral approach focuses on the antecedent conditions or triggers that are likely to set the occasion for the problem behavior and the consequences or effects of the behavior that contribute to maintaining the problem. It is the triggers that lead individuals to drink and it is the effects of alcohol that keep the person drinking. A cycle of alcoholism becomes established. The combination of identifying these triggers and their effects provide a focus for understanding how alcoholism works and for designing interventions to break up the cycle of alcoholism and develop a new cycle of sobriety.

The second perspective is *skill development*. One of the particularly harmful effects of alcoholism is the significant damage individuals experience in critical life skills. Sustained abuse of alcohol impedes, and in more severe cases destroys, an individual's ability to make decisions, take responsibility in daily activities, function socially, and manage their emotions. Personal growth (autonomous, cognitive, social, and emotional) is adversely impacted through alcoholism. Consequently, when individuals become sober, personal skill areas need to be specifically targeted and developed. The position taken in this book is that abstinence from alcohol is not sufficient for a recovering alcoholic to achieve lifelong sobriety. Rather, the combination of abstinence and systematic skill development is needed for recovering alcoholics to achieve lifelong *healthy* sobriety.

These two perspectives are made operational throughout the four sections of the book:

- Section One, Chapters 1–3, addresses information related to understanding the problem of alcohol, developing a behavioral model to explain the cycle of alcoholism and necessary motivational and commitment issues for getting started in a plan to address alcoholism.

- Section Two, Chapters 4–6, describes the relatively universal procedures for disrupting the practice of alcoholism and attaining beginning sobriety.

- Section Three, Chapters 7–11, a critical section in this book, addresses the fundamental and particularly crucial question, "Now that I am sober what's next?" These chapters focus on developing necessary life-skills so that the recovering alcoholic has more opportunity to develop healthy lifelong sobriety. A key assumption is that the recovering alcoholic needs a plan with detailed procedures involving both *abstinence* from alcohol and *skill development* in areas that were substantially impeded or repressed during the individual's period of alcoholism.

- Section Four, Chapters 12 and 13, addresses additional issues related to relapse if the recovering alcoholic resumes drinking and further questions and concerns.

Lifelong Healthy Sobriety

The overall process in helping a person quit consuming alcohol and develop a lifelong practice of healthy sobriety is depicted throughout the book in terms of two pathways. One pathway is designated as the pathway to chronic alcoholism, which the individual followed prior to systematic interventions. The second pathway introduces the alternative, which is a pathway to lifelong, healthy sobriety. The strong implication is that the individual has a choice between maintaining the pathway to chronic alcoholism or, as the title of this book suggests, forging a new pathway to healthy sobriety.

While formidable challenges face alcoholics, their support people, their families and friends, the task is attainable. The how-to for interventions is made accessible. The results have been quite spectacular and inspiring for those who have taken necessary steps to abandon the pathway to alcoholism and to embrace the necessary steps to achieve lifelong sobriety. Unfortunately, there is no quick and easy remedy. There is no silver bullet. Rather, the pathway to healthy sobriety is a daily, lifelong commitment. While the journey is certainly challenging, perhaps daunting for some, the results are immeasurable not only for the individual's family, friends, colleagues, and coworkers but, most of all, for the individuals themselves.

Appendices of Reproducible Forms

APPENDIX A

FORM 3.1: Checklist for Warning Signs of Alcoholism		
Factor	**Applicable** (Underline) **Yes or No** (Maybe is a Yes)	**Explanations of Yes Responses**
1. Do I drink alone when I feel stressed, angry, or depressed?	Yes No	Describe how often:
2. Do I make or find excuses to drink?	Yes No	Name some excuses I use:
3. Does my drinking make me late for work?	Yes No	Describe how often and what happened:
4. Has my family said they are worried about my drinking?	Yes No	Describe what they said or did:
5. Do I drink after telling myself I won't?	Yes No	Describe the most recent example:
6. When I set limits on my drinking, do I fail to keep them?	Yes No	Describe the most recent occurrence:
7. Do I have trouble remembering things I did while drinking?	Yes No	Describe an instance:
8. Do I have headaches, stomach upsets, the shakes, or hangovers the next morning after drinking?	Yes No	Describe ill effects of the most recent example:
9. Do I find I am drinking daily to function?	Yes No	Describe:
10. Do I get angry when confronted about drinking?	Yes No	Describe the last example:
11. Have my eating habits changed much from drinking?	Yes No	Describe in what way they have changed:
12. Am I taking less care of my physical appearance?	Yes No	Describe any changes:
13. Have I had health changes or issues recently?	Yes No	Describe these health issues:
14. Other	Yes No	Explain:
SCORING: Total Number of *Yes* Scores _____ Total Number of *No* Scores _____		
CONCLUSION		
• Score of *Yes* to any item should be addressed. There may be a problem with alcohol. • Score of 2 or more *Yes* items means there most likely is a serious problem with alcohol and help should be obtained (see a doctor and address drinking).		

Source: Adapted from http://www.mysobriety.com/physical_effects.html; http://signsofalcoholism.org.

APPENDIX B

FORM 3.2: Checklist and Action Plan for Committing to Quit Alcohol		
Factor	**Applicable** (underline) **Yes or No**	**Explanation**
1. Have I admitted that I have a drinking problem I cannot control?	Yes No	
2. Have I "bottomed out?"	Yes No	
3. Have I experienced a crisis wake-up call?	Yes No	
4. Have I tried everything to control my drinking and failed?	Yes No	
5. Have I encountered an acquaintance successfully in recovery?	Yes No	
6. Do I have fears about alcohol withdrawal problems?	Yes No	
7. Have family members or close friends intervened with me?	Yes No	
8. Have I closely reviewed the benefits of sobriety?	Yes No	
9. Have I taken graduated steps to self-control?	Yes No	
10. Are there warning signs (From Form 3.1) that I have a drinking problem?	Yes No	
11. Are other warning signs present?	Yes No	

ACTION PLAN

State with reasons what your present decision is regarding making a commitment to quit drinking and undertake a recovery plan.

APPENDIX C

FORM 5.1: Checklist and Action Plan for Cravings

DESCRIPTION OF CRAVINGS

Measurement	Response	Notes
1. Frequency (How often?)		
2. Duration (How long?)		
3. Intensity (How strong?)		

STRATEGIES TO DEFUSE CRAVINGS

Tools	Does this Tool Apply to Me?	Notes
Having the Right Mindset		
1. Knowing what to expect	Yes No	
2 It will get worse before it gets better	Yes No	
3. Expect uncertainty between cravings	Yes No	
4. It too shall pass	Yes No	
5. View cravings as enticements	Yes No	
6. Realize cravings are irrational	Yes No	
Procedures for Defusing Cravings		
1. Contact a friend	Yes No	
2. Get busy	Yes No	
3. Use relaxation strategies	Yes No	
4. Use symbols	Yes No	
5. Think it through	Yes No	
6. Avoid the "cues"	Yes No	
7. Planned escapes	Yes No	

ACTION PLAN

APPENDIX D

FORM 6.1: Checklist and Action Plan for Initial Needs		
Item	**Selection (Underline)**	**Notes**
Preparing Oneself Beforehand	Yes No	
Filling the Void with Constructive Practices	Yes No	
Taking Care of One's Physical-Well Being	Yes No	
Sleep	Yes No	
Diet	Yes No	
Personal Hygiene and Appearance	Yes No	
Living with Diminished Life Skills	Yes No	
Establishing Support		
Support Groups –Meetings	Yes No	
Personal Support	Yes No	
Dealing with the Pressures to Drink	Yes No	
Drinking Locations	Yes No	
"Drinking Buddies"	Yes No	
Parties and Gatherings	Yes No	
Avoiding the Trouble Spots	Yes No	
Managing Alcohol Rituals	Yes No	
Keeping a Journal	Yes No	
Other	Yes No	

ACTION PLAN

The main parts of my action plan to begin with are:

APPENDIX E

FORM 8.1: Procedural Steps for Developing Routines
Step 1: Pinpoint a difficult responsibility and get started.
Step 2: Write down how this responsibility is usually handled.
Step 3: Write down a specific routine for this period.
Step 4: Adapt the routine as necessary.
Step 5: Implement the routine for three consecutive days.
Step 6: Evaluate the effectiveness of the routine.
Step 7: Plan for other areas of responsibilities.

APPENDIX F

FORM 8.2: Procedural Steps for Solving Problems Effectively
Step 1: Recognize the problem.
Step 2: Clarify the problem.
Step 3: Identify explanations for the problem.
Step 4: List intervention options.
Step 5: Select the most favorable option.
Step 6: Implement intervention.
Step 7: Evaluate effectiveness.
Step 8: Decide to maintain, modify, or change intervention.

APPENDIX G

FORM 8.3: Planning Guide for Managing To-Do Lists					
Step 1 To-Do List List tasks to be done	Step 2 Priority (Underline) 1: Somewhat Important 2: Important 3: Very Important	Step 3 Scheduled for (Underline) 1: Short Task 2: Medium task 3: Long task	Step 4 Completed (Underline) Yes or No	Step 5 Rescheduled for	Step 6 Review Note any explanations, successes, decisions, or insights
	1　2　3	1　2　3 Date: Time:	Yes　No	Date: Time:	
	1　2　3	1　2　3 Date: Time:	Yes　No	Date: Time:	
	1　2　3	1　2　3 Date: Time:	Yes　No	Date: Time:	
	1　2　3	1　2　3 Date: Time:	Yes　No	Date: Time:	
	1　2　3	1　2　3 Date: Time:	Yes　No	Date: Time:	
	1　2　3	1　2　3 Date: Time:	Yes　No	Date: Time:	
	1　2　3	1　2　3 Date: Time:	Yes　No	Date: Time:	
	1　2　3	1　2　3 Date: Time:	Yes　No	Date: Time:	

APPENDIX H

FORM 8.4: Checklist and Action Plan for Coping Skills		
Skill	Selection (Underline)	Notes
Assessing the problem situation:		
• Problem is uncontrollable and unchangeable.	Yes No	
• Situation can be left.	Yes No	
Problem situation accepted	Yes No	
Manage the moment		
• Use self-talk	Yes No	
• Focus on one aspect of task	Yes No	
• Use breaks	Yes No	
• Understand "it too shall pass"	Yes No	
• Other	Yes No	
Restore the balance		
• Take a walk	Yes No	
• Work out at the gym	Yes No	
• Gardening	Yes No	
• Listen to/play music	Yes No	
• Read a popular book/magazine	Yes No	
• Surf the net	Yes No	
• Shopping	Yes No	
• Relaxation breathing	Yes No	
• Yoga	Yes No	
• Meditation	Yes No	
• Hobbies	Yes No	
• Take a class	Yes No	
• Other	Yes No	
ACTION PLAN		

APPENDIX I

FORM 9.1: Checklist and Action Plan for Memory Loss		
Step 1: Identify the Signs of Memory Loss	Selection (Underline) Yes or No	Notes
1. Loss of recall	Yes No	
2. Easily distracted	Yes No	
3. Preoccupation	Yes No	
4. Short attention span	Yes No	
5. Difficulty planning and following plans	Yes No	
6. Difficulty in completing routines	Yes No	
7. Misplacing items	Yes No	
8. Difficulty in making conversation	Yes No	
9. Forgetting familiar routines	Yes No	
10. Other	Yes No	
Results for Step 1 Total Number of *Yes* Scores _____		
A. 6 or more *Yes* items selected	Yes No	Significant problems
B. 3–5 *Yes* items selected	Yes No	Some problems
C. 1–2 *Yes* items selected	Yes No	Minimal problems
Step 2: Take Concrete Steps to Enhance the Memory Faculty		
1. Write it down	Yes No	
2. Use visual cues	Yes No	
3. Have set place for frequently used items	Yes No	
4. Use repetition	Yes No	

APPENDIX I

FORM 9.1 *Continued*		
5. Engage in memory-based brain games	Yes No	
6. Establish routines	Yes No	
7. Stimulate the mind	Yes No	
8. Physical exercise	Yes No	
9. Other	Yes No	
ACTION PLAN (Combining Steps 1 and 2)		

APPENDIX J

FORM 9.2: Checklist and Action Plan for Faulty Thinking Patterns		
Step 1: Identify the Destructive Thinking Patterns	Selection (Underline) Yes or No	Notes
1. Inability to make decisions	Yes No	
2. Grandiosity	Yes No	
3. Judgmentalism	Yes No	
4. Intolerance	Yes No	
5. Manipulative	Yes No	
6. Self-centered	Yes No	
7. Dishonest	Yes No	
8. Impulsivity and instant gratification	Yes No	
9. False attribution	Yes No	
10. Victim-entitlement cycle	Yes No	
11. Obsessing	Yes No	
12. Other	Yes No	
Results for Step 1 Total Number of *Yes* Scores _____	Selection (Underline)	Notes
A. 6 or more items *Yes* selected	Yes No	
B. 3–5 *Yes* items selected	Yes No	
C. 1–2 *Yes* items selected	Yes No	
Step 2: Build Constructive Thinking Skills		
1. Learn from meetings	Yes No	
2. Learn from sponsor or support person	Yes No	
3. Learn from professional help	Yes No	

APPENDIX J

FORM 9.2 *Continued*

4. Learn from journaling and reflecting	Yes No	
5. Learn from significant people	Yes No	
6. Learn from classes	Yes No	
7. Reject negative thinking	Yes No	
8. Other	Yes No	

ACTION PLAN

APPENDIX K

FORM 10.1: Rating Scale for Impact of Social Deficiencies		
Crucial Life Areas	**Rating of Impact** (Underline) 0—No impact 1—Some impact 2—Serious impact	**Notes**
1. Employment (At risk? Written up? Warned?)	0 1 2	
2. Relationships (Have friends? Go to gatherings? Meet?)	0 1 2	
3. Alienation (Rejected? Left out?)	0 1 2	
4. Loneliness (Feel the pain or pinch? Brood? Worry about being alone?)	0 1 2	
5. Problem solving (Fix things? Talk things through?)	0 1 2	
6. Other (for example, Awareness)	0 1 2	
Results Total Score _____	**Selection**	**Notes**
A. Score of 6 or more	Yes No	Full social competence intervention needed
B. Score between 2 and 5	Yes No	Some intervention needed
C. Score less than 2	Yes No	No intervention needed
DECISION		

APPENDIX L

FORM 10.2: Rating Scale for Social Competence

Social Competency	Rating (Underline) 0—Not applicable 1—Somewhat applicable 2—Very applicable	Social Deficiency	Notes
1. Honesty	2 1 0 1 2	1. Dishonesty	
2. Empathetic	2 1 0 1 2	2. Insensitive	
3. Remorseful	2 1 0 1 2	3. Unrepentant	
4. Peaceful	2 1 0 1 2	4. Aggressive	
5. Problem solves	2 1 0 1 2	5. Blames others	
6. Calm	2 1 0 1 2	6. Angry & irritable	
7. Controlled	2 1 0 1 2	7. Impulsive	
8. Responsible	2 1 0 1 2	8. Irresponsible	
9. Responsive	2 1 0 1 2	9. Non-responsive	
10. Attentive to others	2 1 0 1 2	10. Self-centered	
11. Communicates	2 1 0 1 2	11. Miscommunicates	
12. Follows procedures	2 1 0 1 2	12. Non-complies	
13. Sexually appropriate	2 1 0 1 2	13. Promiscuous	
	1 2 **Danger Zone**		

Results: List Items Scoring 1 or 2 in Social Deficiency Direction (Danger Zone)

Items Scored 2	Items Scored 1

DECISION

APPENDIX M

FORM 10.3: Checklist and Action Plan for Developing Social Competence		
Strategies for Developing Social Competence	**Selection** (Underline) Yes or No	**Notes**
1. Active reflection	Yes No	
2. Ongoing feedback from support person	Yes No	
3. Attendance at meetings and related social gatherings	Yes No	
4. Engaging in service work	Yes No	
5. Modeling from significant persons	Yes No	
6. Stepping out and taking measured risks	Yes No	
7. Understanding and maintaining relationships	Yes No	
8. Addressing sexual relationships	Yes No	
9. Using self-help instruction	Yes No	
10. Seeking professional help	Yes No	
ACTION PLAN		

APPENDIX N

FORM 11.1: Checklist for Determining Target Emotions			
Positive Emotions	**Selection** (Underline) Yes or No	**Negative Emotions**	**Selection** (Underline)
1. Joyful: happy, excited, exhilarant, jubilant, merry, exalted, cheer, glad, elated, proud	Yes No	**1. Fearful:** afraid, frightened, terrified, threatened, insecure	Yes No
2. Loving: love, affection, care, compassion, kind, generous. courageous	Yes No	**2. Angry:** hateful, fury, irritable, rage, resentment, antipathy, offended, disgusted, annoyed	Yes No
3. Peaceful: comfortable, serene, mellow, relish, calm, fulfilled, satisfied, modest, humble	Yes No	**3. Anxious:** dismayed, distressed, perturbed, worried, frustrated, edgy, needful	Yes No
4. Hopeful: hope, optimism, desiring, wanting, goal directed, needful.	Yes No	**4. Depressed:** hopeless, despair, discouraged, disheartened, miserable, morbid, apathy, boredom, sadness, despondent, disappointed	Yes No
5. Grateful: thankful, gratitude, appreciative	Yes No	**5.Self-Pity:** pained, injured, sick, tired, excuses, envy, jealousy, lonliness, alone, rejected	Yes No
Positive Emotions Results Prioritize No Selections (1 or 2 only) 1. 2.		**Negative Emotions Results** Prioritize Yes Selections (1 or 2 only) 3. 4.	

APPENDIX O

FORM 11.2: Checklist for Determining Operating Triggers		
Prioritized List of Positive Emotions from Form 11.1 1. 2..		Prioritized List of Negative Emotions from Form 11.1 3. 4.

Triggers	**Selection** (Underline)	**Notes**
1. Thoughts	Yes No	
2. Communication	Yes No	
3. Reminders or flashbacks	Yes No	
4. Unresolved conflicts	Yes No	
5. Breakdown in relationships	Yes No	
6. Adapting to changes	Yes No	
7. Making decisions	Yes No	
8. Impact of environment	Yes No	
9. Health issues	Yes No	
10. Marginal living	Yes No	
11. Victim dispositions	Yes No	
12. Social ineptness	Yes No	
13. Personal issues	Yes No	
14. Personal safety	Yes No	
15. Other	Yes No	

RESULTS: Prioritize Yes Selections (2 or 3) Operating Triggers

1.
2.
3.

APPENDIX P

FORM 11.3: Checklist and Action Plan for Developing Emotional Growth

Prioritized Emotions from Form 11.1		Operating Triggers from Form 11.2
1. 2.	3. 4.	1. 2. 3. .

Strategies	Selection (Underline) Yes or No	Specifics
1. Maintain initial strategies for obtaining sobriety	Yes No	
2. Utilize strategies for developing autonomous growth	Yes No	
3. Utilize strategies for developing cognitive growth	Yes No	
4. Utilize strategies for developing social growth	Yes No	
5. Engage in service activities	Yes No	
6. Manage the triggers for negative emotions	Yes No	
7. Manage the triggers for positive emotions	Yes No	
8. Use coping skills for triggers	Yes No	
9. Enhance positive emotions	Yes No	
10. Reduce destructive negative thoughts	Yes No	
11. Increase constructive positive thoughts	Yes No	
12. Adopt meditation practice	Yes No	
13 Establish replacement behaviors	Yes No	
14. Other	Yes No	

ACTION PLAN

APPENDIX Q

FORM 12.1: Checklist and Action Plan for Preventing Future Relapse

Contributing Factors to Relapse	Applicability Rating (Underline) Yes: Applicable No: Not applicable	General Strategies (from Box 12.2)
1. Treating relapse as part of recovery	Yes No	Avoid relapse at all costs with a comprehensive recovery plan.
2. The nature of addiction and disease	Yes No	Re-examine alcoholism as an addiction-disease.
3. Interacting effects of alcoholism	Yes No	Re-examine the damaging effects of alcoholism.
4. Inadequate planning in the first place	Yes No	Develop a comprehensive plan from quitting to healthy sobriety.
5. Abandonment of effective practices	Yes No	Pick up previously used effective practices used following detoxification.
6. Need to test the waters	Yes No	Avoid this at all costs. But if insistent ensure full return to recovery plan if problems arise.
7. The reinforcement–extinction cycle	Yes No	Recognize the role of support from others but fully invest in your own efforts.
8. Managing surprises or extenuating circumstances	Yes No	There are no exceptions. Never take a drink.
9. Edging closer to former haunts and routines	Yes No	Make a firm resolve to avoid situations where drinking is likely.
10. Seeking just cause	Yes No	Recognize this is denial. Make the firm resolve to quit and stay sober.

SUMMARY

Factors scored Yes:
Underline and total: 1 2 3 4 5 6 7 8 9 10   Total Yes: _____
Factors scored No: Total No: _____

ACTION PLAN (Select strategies to match the contributing factors scored Yes).

References

Alcoholics Anonymous. (2001). *Alcoholics anonymous* (The Big Book, 3rd ed.). New York: Alcoholics Anonymous World Services.

Alcoholics Anonymous. (2008). *Twelve steps and twelve traditions* (14th ed.). New York: Alcoholics Anonymous World Services.

Alcoholics Anonymous, AA On-line Forum: http://stinkin-thinkin.com/2009/03/23/dry-drunk/

Alderfer, C. P. (1972). *Existence, relatedness, and growth: Human needs in organizational settings.* Glencoe, IL: Free Press

Bates, M. E., Bowden, S. C., & Barry, D. (2002). Neurocognitive impairment associated with alcohol use disorders: Implications for treatment. *Experimental and Clinical Psychopharmacology, 10*(3), 193–212.

Beck, J. S. (1995). *Cognitive therapy: Basics and beyond.* New York: Guilford Press.

Big Book Concordance. (n.d.). www.royy.com/concord.html, retrieved 11/24/10

Bill W. (1988). *The language of the heart: Bill W's grapevine writings.* New York: AA Grapevine.

Billig, M. (1999). *Freudian repression: Conversation creating the unconscious.* New York: Cambridge University Press.

Boud, D., Keogh, R., & Walker, D. (1985). *Reflection: Turning experience into learning.* New York: Routledge.

Broe, G. A., Creasey, H., Jorm, A. F., Bennett, H. P., Casey, B., Waite, L. M., Grayson, D. A., & Cullen, J. (2008). Health habits and risk of cognitive impairment and dementia in old age: A prospective study on the effects of exercise, smoking, and alcohol consumption. *Australian and New Zealand Journal of Public Health, 22*(5), 621–623.

Burton, G., & Dimbleby, R. (2006). *Between ourselves: An introduction to interpersonal communication* (3rd ed.). Soho Square, London, UK: Bloomsbury.

Carr, J., & Wilder, D. A. (2004). *Functional assessment and intervention: A guide to understanding behavior* (2nd ed.). Homewood, IL: High Tide Press.

Chodron, P. (1997). *When things fall apart: Heart advice for difficult times.* Boston, MA: Shambhala Publications.

Colvin, G. (1999). *Defusing anger and aggression: Safe strategies for secondary school educators* (Video/DVD program). Eugene, OR: Iris Media.

Colvin, G. (2004). *Managing the cycle of acting-out behavior in the classroom.* Eugene, OR: Behavior Associates.

Colvin, G. (2008). *Managing the cycle of emotional escalation.* In R. Sprick & M. Garrison (Eds.), *Interventions: Evidence-based behavioral strategies of individual students* (2nd ed.) (pp. 425–462). Eugene, OR: Pacific Northwest Publishing.

Colvin, G. (2009). *Managing noncompliance and defiance in the classroom: A road map for teachers, specialists, and behavior support teams.* Thousand Oaks, CA: Corwin.

Colvin, G. (2010). *Defusing disruptive behavior in the classroom.* Thousand Oaks, CA: Corwin.

Colvin, G., & Sheehan, M. (2012). *Managing the cycle of meltdowns for students with autism spectrum disorder.* Thousand Oaks, CA: Corwin.

Contreras, D. A. (2010). *Psychology of thinking (Psychology of emotions, motivations and actions).* New York: Nova Science.

Cooper, J. O., Heron, T. E., & Heward, W. L. (2007). *Applied behavior analysis* (2nd ed.). Upper Saddle River, NJ: Pearson Education.

Coulter, D., Coulter, J., & Coulter, D. (2005). *Manners for the real world: Basic social skills.* Winston-Salem, NC: Coulter Video.

Cyster, E. (2008). *Teach yourself etiquette and modern manners.* Blacklick, OH: McGraw-Hill.

Davis, M., Robbins, E., McKay, M., & Fanning, P. (2008). *The relaxation & stress reduction workbook (New-Harbinger self-help workbook).* Oakland, CA: New Harbinger Publications.

Dean, H. (2010). *Understanding human need.* Bristol, U.K.: Policy Press.

Edwards, G., & Lader, M. (1994). *Addiction: Processes of Change.* New York: Oxford University Press.

Elliott, R. (2001). *Self confidence trainer.* Argyll, Scotland: Uncommon Knowledge LLP.

Ellis, A. (2001). *Overcoming destructive beliefs, feelings, and behaviors: new directions for rational emotive behavior therapy.* Buffalo, NY: Prometheus Books.

Fein, G., Bachman, L., Fisher, S., & Davenport, L. (1990). Cognitive impairments in abstinent alcoholics. *Addiction Medicine, 152,* 531–537.

Fernandez-Serrano, M. J., Lozano, O., Perez-Garcia, M., & Verdejo-Garcia, A. (2010). Impact of severity of drug use on discrete emotions recognition in polysubstance abusers. *Drug and Alcohol Dependence, 109,* 57–64.

Fontana, D. (1994). *Social skills at work (Problems in practice series).* New York: Routledge, Chapman, & Hall.

Fox, S. (2002). *Etiquette survival: Dining and social skills for adults and teens.* Los Gatos, CA: Etiquette Survival.

Frankl, V. (1983). *Man's search for meaning* (3rd ed.). New York: Simon & Schuster.

Gallagher, W. (1993). *The power of place.* New York: Poseiden Press.

Geoff C., & Scott W. (April 2011). The Challenge of the 11th Step: Sustaining the practice of meditation: Part I, Why meditate? *Emerald Valley Intergroup Newsletter,* pp. 1, 3, 7.

Geoff C., & Scott W. (July 2011). The Challenge of the 11th Step: Sustaining the practice of meditation: Part II, Some guidelines for meditation. *Emerald Valley Intergroup Newsletter,* pp. 1, 5.

Goleman, D. (1995). *Emotional intelligence.* New York: Bantam Books

Gorski, T. T. (1989). *Passages through recovery—An action plan for preventing elapse.* Center City, MN: Hazelden, 1989.

Gorski, T. T., & Miller, M. (1986). *Staying sober: A guide for relapse prevention.* Independence, MO: Herald House/Independence Press.

Greenberg, J. (1964). *I never promised you a rose garden.* New York: Henry Holt & Company.

Greenfield, G. (1984). *We need each other: Deeper levels in our interpersonal relationships.* Grand Rapids, MI: Baker Publishing Group.

Harper, C. (1988). The pathology of alcohol-related brain damage: An overview. *Australian Drug and Alcohol Review, 7*(1), 51–55.

Hertnon, S. (2005). *Theory of universal human needs.* Auckland, N.Z.: Nakedize Publishing.

Herzberg, F. (1959). *The motivation to work.* New York: John Wiley and Sons.

Jellinek, E. M. (1960). *The disease concept of alcoholism.* New Haven, CT: Hillhouse.

Kelly, A. (2007). *Social skills and communication consultancy.* www.alexkelly.biz/

Kelly, M. (2007). *The seven levels of intimacy: The art of loving and the joy of being loved.* New York: Fireside.

Ketcham, K., Asbury, W. F., Schulstad, M., & Ciaramicoli, A. P. (2000). *Beyond the influence: Understanding and defeating alcoholism.* New York: Bantam Books.

Malouf, J. M., & Schutte, N. S. (2007). *Activities to enhance social, emotional, and problem-solving skills: Seventy-six activities that teach children, adolescents, and adults skills crucial to success in life.* Springfield, IL: Charles Thomas.

Maslow, A. (1954). *Motivation and personality.* New York: Harper and Row.

Martinic, M., & Leigh, B. (2004). *Reasonable risk-alcohol in perspective.* New York: Brunner-Routledge.

McCoy, K. (2007). *Alcoholics have trouble reading others' emotions.* Alcoholism: Clinical & Experimental Research, news release, Feb. 22, 2007. http://health.msn.com/health-topics/mental-health/articlepage.aspx?cp-documentid=100156672; retrieved 11/19/10.

McGinnis, E., & Goldstein, A. P. (2003). *Skillstreaming in early childhood: New strategies for teaching prosocial social skills* (Rev. ed.). Champaign, IL: Research Press.

McKee, A., Boyatz, R., & Johnston, F. (2008). *Becoming a resonant leader: Develop your emotional intelligence, renew your relationships, sustain your effectiveness.* Boston, MA: Harvard Business School Publishing.

Medina, J. (2008). *Brain rules: 12 principles for surviving and thriving at work, home, and school.* Seattle, WA: Pear Press.

Michie, D. (2008). *Hurry up and meditate: Your starter kit for inner peace and better health.* Crows Nest, Australia: Allen & Unwin.

Monti, P. M., Abrams, D. B., Kadden, R. M., & Cooney, N. L. (1989). *Treating Alcohol Dependence: A Coping Skills Training Guide.* New York: Guilford.

Morgenstern, J., & Longabaugh, R. (2000). Cognitive-behavioral treatment for alcohol dependence: a review of evidence for its hypothesized mechanisms of action. *Addiction, 95,* 1475–1490.

National Institute on Alcohol Abuse and Alcoholism (NIAAA). (n.d.). *Alcohol problems in intimate relationships: Identification and intervention.* http://pubs.niaaa.nih.gov/publications/niaaa-guide/NIAAA_AAMF_%20Final.pdf.

National Institute on Alcohol Abuse and Alcoholism. (2003). *Underage drinking, a major public health challenge.* pubs.niaaa.nih.gov/publications/aa59.htm

Nelson, B. B. (2007). *The emotion code: How to release your trapped emotions for abundant health, love, and happiness.* Mesquite, NV: Wellness Unmasked Publishing.

Oltmanns, T. F., & Emery, R. E. (2010). *Abnormal psychology* (6th ed.). Upper Saddle River, NJ: Prentice Hall.

Ortony, A., & Turner, T. J. (1990). What's basic about emotions? *Psychological Review, 97,* 315–331.

Parrot, W. (2001). *Emotions in Social Psychology.* Philadelphia, PA: Psychology Press

Patterson, G. R., & Forgatch, M. S. (2005). *Parents and adolescents living together: The basics* (2nd ed.). Champaign, IL: Research Press.

Plutchik, R. (1980). A general psychoevolutionary theory of emotion. In R. Plutchik & H. Kellerman (Eds.), *Emotion: Theory, research, and experience: Vol. 1. Theories of emotion* (pp. 3–33). New York: Academic Press.

Polivy, J., & Herman, C. P. (2002). If at first you don't succeed: False hopes of self-change. *American Psychologist, 57,* 677–689.

Quigley, B., Leonard, K., & Collins, R. (2003). Characteristics of violent bars and bar patrons. *Journal of Studies of Alcohol, 64,* 765–772.

Rosenbloom, M. J., Pfefferbaum, A., & Sullivan, E. V. (1995). Structural brain alterations associated with alcoholism. *Alcohol Health & Research World, 19*(4), 266–272.

Rosenfeld, P., Culbertson, A. L., & Magnusson, P. (1992). *Human needs: A literature review and cognitive life span model.* Report presented to the Navy Personnel Research and Development Center, San Diego, CA.

Roy Y. (1997). *The big book concordance.* New York: Alcoholics Anonymous World Services. http://www.royy.com/ab.html

Saggers, S., & Gray, D. (1998). *Dealing with alcohol: Indigenous usage in Australia, New Zealand, and Canada.* Cambridge, UK: Cambridge University Press.

Scribner, R. A., MacKinnon, D. P., & Dwyer, J. H. (1995). The risk of assaultive violence and alcohol availability in Los Angeles County. *American Journal of Public Health, 85,* 335–340.

Simerson, B. K., & McCormick, M. D. (2003). *Fired, laid off, out of a job: A manual for understanding, coping, surviving.* Westport, CT: Praeger.

Sober Recovery Community. (2009). [Website]. www.soberrecovery.com/forums/alcoholism/83300-what-alcoholic-thinking.html

Solberg, R. J. (1983). *The dry drunk syndrome.* Center City, MN: Hazelden.

Steel, P. (2007). The nature of procrastination: A meta-analytic and theoretical review of quintessential self-regulatory failure. *Psychological Bulletin, 133*(1), 65–94.

Townsend, J. M., & Duka, T. (2003). Mixed emotions: Impairments in the recognition of specific emotional facial expressions. *Neuropsychologia, 41,* 773–782.

Twelve Steps and Twelve Traditions (14th ed.). (2008). New York: Alcoholics Anonymous World Services.

U.S. Department of Health and Human Services, Substance Abuse and Mental Health Services Administration. (2002, September 4). Results from the 2001 National Household Survey on Drug Abuse: Volume I. Summary of National Findings. Office of Applied Studies, NHSDA Series H-17 ed. (BKD461, SMA 02-3758) Washington, DC: www.oas.samhsa.gov/nhsda/2k1nhsda/vol1/Chapter3.htm

Vaillant, G. E. (1995). *The natural history of alcoholism revisited.* Cambridge, MA: Harvard.

Vrajaprana, P. (1999). *Vedanta: A simple introduction.* Hollywood, CA: Vedanta Press.

Washton, A. M., & Zweben, J. E. (2006). *Treating Alcohol and Drug Problems in Psycho-therapy* Practice. New York: Guilford Press.

White, A. M. (2003). What happened? Alcohol, memory, blackouts, and the brain. *Alcohol Research & Health, 27*(2), 186–196.

Witkiewitz, K. & Marlatt, G. A. (2009). Relapse prevention for alcohol and drug problems: That was Zen, this is Tao. In G. A. Marlatt & K. Witkiewitz (Eds.), *Addictive behaviors: New readings on etiology, prevention, and treatment* (pp. 403–427). Washington, DC: American Psychological Association.

Index

Page references followed by *f* indicate figures.

R

S